Advanced Clinical Technologies in Treating Neurosurgical Diseases

Advanced Clinical Technologies in Treating Neurosurgical Diseases

Guest Editors

Franco Servadei
Kenan Arnautovic
Roberto Stefini

MDPI

Basel • Beijing • Wuhan • Barcelona • Belgrade • Novi Sad • Cluj • Manchester

Guest Editors
Franco Servadei
Global Neurosurgery
Programme Fondazione
IRCCS
Istituto Neurologico Carlo
Besta
Milan
Italy

Kenan Arnautovic
Semmes-Murphey Clinic
University of Tennessee
Memphis
USA

Roberto Stefini
Department of Neurosurgery
Legnano Hospital
Milan
Italy

Editorial Office
MDPI AG
Grosspeteranlage 5
4052 Basel, Switzerland

This is a reprint of the Special Issue, published open access by the journal *Brain Sciences* (ISSN 2076-3425), freely accessible at: https://www.mdpi.com/journal/brainsci/special_issues/OCVN990G86.

For citation purposes, cite each article independently as indicated on the article page online and as indicated below:

Lastname, A.A.; Lastname, B.B. Article Title. *Journal Name* **Year**, *Volume Number*, Page Range.

ISBN 978-3-7258-5339-7 (Hbk)
ISBN 978-3-7258-5340-3 (PDF)
https://doi.org/10.3390/books978-3-7258-5340-3

Contents

Contents

brain sciences

MDPI

Editorial

Multidisciplinary Innovation in Neurosurgery and Neuroscience: Advancing Frontiers in Diagnosis, Therapy, and Neurological Rehabilitation

Delia Cannizzaro [1], Roberto Stefini [1], Kenan Arnautovic [2] and Franco Servadei [3,*]

1 Department of Neurosurgery, ASST Ovest Milano Legnano Hospital, Legnano, 20025 Milan, Italy; delia.cannizzaro@gmail.com (D.C.)
2 Semmes Murphey Clinic and Department of Neurosurgery, University of Tennessee, Memphis, TN 38163, USA; kenanarnaut@yahoo.com
3 Global Neurosurgery Programme Fondazione IRCCS Istituto Neurologico Carlo Besta, 20133 Milan, Italy
* Correspondence: franco.servadei@gmail.com

In recent years, neurosurgery and clinical neuroscience have undergone a profound transformation, driven by an increasingly interdisciplinary approach that integrates technological innovation, the refinement of therapeutic protocols, and novel rehabilitative paradigms [1]. These advances are reshaping the management of complex neurological disorders and promoting the development of more effective, less invasive, and highly personalized treatment strategies [2].

This Special Issue of *Brain Sciences* presents nine original contributions that collectively illustrate the breadth and depth of these transformative innovations. The studies featured span topics from minimally invasive spinal surgery and advanced neurosurgical training to intraoperative fluorescence-guided resection, nanomedicine-based drug delivery, and invasive brain–computer interfaces (BCIs), offering a multifaceted yet cohesive vision of the future of neurosurgery.

The adoption of 3D navigation systems is enhancing surgical outcomes by minimizing reliance on traditional instruments, paving the way for more precise and less invasive procedures. In the context of spinal surgery, Bielecki et al. (Contribution 1) demonstrated the clinical utility of the Single-Step Pedicle Screw System (SSPSS) combined with three-dimensional neuronavigation. By eliminating the need for a K-wire and standardizing optimal screw trajectories, the authors achieved a high accuracy rate (95%) in pedicle screw placement and a significant reduction in intraoperative complications. This approach represents a substantial evolution toward safer and more reproducible minimally invasive spinal procedures. In the same way, intraoperative CT-based navigation significantly improves the safety and precision of posterior fixation in congenital craniovertebral junction anomalies, enabling tailored surgical strategies that avoid neurovascular injury and eliminate the need for more invasive hardware, thus representing a meaningful advancement in complex spinal neurosurgery (Contribution 2).

The use of Virtual iMRI in combination with intraoperative imaging represents a promising advance in brain tumor surgery. Grasso et al. (2025) evaluated the elastic image fusion (EIF) method, which combines preoperative MRI with intraoperative CT to better detect residual tumors during glioblastoma surgery. Virtual iMRI showed high sensitivity (100%) but lower specificity (50%), while intraoperative CT had lower sensitivity (56%) but perfect specificity (Contribution 3).

The field of medical education has also embraced immersive technologies. Guerrini et al. (2024) report that the use of augmented reality (AR) and hands-on simulation significantly improves early neurosurgical training. Virtual learning environments not only increase student engagement, they also enhance preoperative technical skills in a controlled, risk-free setting, bridging the gap between theoretical knowledge and clinical competence (Contribution 4).

Fluorescence-guided surgery continues to refine the precision of brain tumor resections. Alomari et al. (2024) investigated the intraoperative use of sodium fluorescein (SF) in vestibular schwannoma surgery, showing that it facilitates extensive tumor resection while minimizing perioperative morbidity. This technique represents a valuable adjunct for maximizing oncological clearance while preserving neurological function (Contribution 5).

New small devices are also being employed for applications in the operating room: non-penetrating titanium clips represent an effective and safe alternative to traditional sutures for dural closure in intradural spinal surgeries, significantly reducing cerebrospinal fluid leak rates and preserving dural integrity, while also minimizing operative time and imaging artifacts (Contribution 6).

In neurovascular surgery, the emergence of new endovascular devices has enabled the treatment of increasingly complex aneurysms. Jee et al. (2024) highlight the clinical efficacy of flow-diverting stents, reporting high aneurysm occlusion rates and a progressive reduction in periprocedural complications. These findings underscore the importance of technical maturation and patient-specific evaluation in the management of cerebrovascular pathologies (Contribution 7).

Robotic-assisted surgery represents another transformative frontier in neurosurgical practice, particularly in the domain of microsurgical precision. Four major robotic platforms—Symani, Da Vinci, ZEUS, and MUSA—widely used in surgical practice were explored across 48 studies involving vascular, lymphatic, and neural anastomoses. While the initial procedural times were longer than those for manual techniques, the analysis demonstrated a clear trend toward improved efficiency as surgical teams progressed along the learning curve. Importantly, the review highlights the potential for robotic systems to enhance neurovascular procedures, particularly in delicate tasks such as microsuturing for bypass surgery [3,4].

A key contribution by Khan et al. (2025) presents a scoping review on invasive BCIs aimed at restoring communication in patients with severe motor deficits, such as those resulting from ALS, brainstem stroke, or high cervical spinal cord injury. Recent advances in intracortical neural decoding—translating brain signals into text or synthesized speech—offer a therapeutic frontier with the potential to restore communicative autonomy in otherwise locked-in patients. These innovations represent a foundational milestone in neurotechnological rehabilitation (Contribution 8).

Nanotechnology is also opening up new therapeutic pathways in neuro-oncology. Khilar et al. (2025) reviewed strategies employing engineered nanoparticles for the targeted delivery of chemotherapeutic, immunotherapeutic, and radiotherapeutic agents. By enhancing blood–brain barrier permeability and enabling combined treatment modalities (e.g., radio-immunotherapy), these nanocarriers hold great promise for overcoming existing pharmacologic limitations. However, the transition to clinical application necessitates further investigations into long-term safety and nanotoxicology (Contribution 9).

Collectively, these studies demonstrate that neurosurgery is no longer an isolated specialty but rather a convergence point for biomedical engineering, computational neuroscience, advanced simulation-based education, and translational oncology. Emerging technologies—from neuronavigation and intraoperative fluorescence to BCIs and nanomedicine—are not only improving clinical outcomes but fundamentally redefining the paradigms of diagnosis, intervention, and rehabilitation.

To consolidate these promising advances and ensure their widespread adoption, future efforts must prioritize multicenter prospective trials, regulatory validation, and economic sustainability. Nevertheless, the momentum in this field is undeniable.

Neurosurgery and neuroscience are entering a phase of rapid transformation. The integration of advanced technologies—from implantable devices and AR simulators to precision nanotherapeutics—is enhancing not only therapeutic interventions but also medical training and patients' quality of life. Innovations such as flow diversion and fluorescein-guided surgery place surgical precision and safety at the heart of clinical progress, while immersive simulation is revolutionizing professional training. In parallel, invasive BCIs offer a tangible hope of restoring essential functions such as communication in patients otherwise rendered voiceless. Nanomedicine, meanwhile, appears poised to overcome longstanding pharmacological barriers in the treatment of brain tumors, although robust clinical validation remains essential. These findings underscore the value of robotic technologies in extending the boundaries of technical feasibility and precision in cranial neurosurgery and merit further clinical validation and the integration of robotics into advanced neurovascular interventions.

Artificial intelligence is rapidly emerging as a pivotal tool in neurosurgery, enhancing diagnostic accuracy, surgical planning, and intraoperative decision-making through advanced data analysis and machine learning algorithms. Predictive models developed using AI can stratify patient risk, anticipate surgical outcomes, and personalize treatment strategies, promoting evidence-based precision neurosurgery [5–7].

Ultimately, the synergy between technology, surgery, and neuroscience holds the potential to transform complex neurological disease management, from optimizing minimally invasive procedures to revolutionizing specialist training and pioneering new oncologic and rehabilitative strategies. This multidisciplinary convergence, anchored in both technological innovation and clinical insights, promises a future in which neurosciences will not only advance therapies but fundamentally reshape our understanding and treatment of neurological disease.

In reflecting on this progress, it is worth recalling the metaphor coined by Bernard of Chartres in the 12th century, often invoked in medicine, to acknowledge our intellectual debt to the giants on whose shoulders we stand: our earlier inspirations. While that legacy remains foundational, it is increasingly complemented by the transformative role of emerging technologies, which continue to empower us to elevate the standard of care for our patients.

Author Contributions: Conceptualization, F.S. and K.A.; methodology, D.C.; software, D.C.; validation, R.S., F.S. and K.A.; formal analysis, D.C.; investigation, R.S.; resources, R.S.; data curation, D.C.; writing—original draft preparation, D.C.; writing—review and editing, F.S.; visualization, K.A.; supervision, F.S.; project administration, R.S.; funding acquisition, F.S. All authors have read and agreed to the published version of the manuscript.

Conflicts of Interest: The authors have no conflicts of interest, except for Franco Servadei, who reports grant and consultancy fees from Finceramica Integra INTA.

List of Contributions

1. Bielecki, M.; Boadi, B.I.; Xie, Y.; Ikwuegbuenyi, C.A.; Farooq, M.; Berger, J.; Hernández-Hernández, A.; Hussain, I.; Härtl, R. High Accuracy of Three-Dimensional Navigated Kirschner-Wire-Less Single-Step Pedicle Screw System (SSPSS) in Lumbar Fusions: Comparison of Intraoperatively Planned versus Final Screw Position. *Brain Sci.* **2024**, *14*, 873. https://doi.org/10.3390/brainsci14090873.
2. Cracchiolo, G.; Baram, A.; Capo, G.; Rossini, Z.; Riva, A.; Fanti, A.; De Robertis, M.; Fornari, M.; Pessina, F.; Brembilla, C. The Impact of Intraoperative CT-Based Navigation in Congenital

Craniovertebral Junction Anomalies: New Concepts of Treatment. *Brain Sci.* **2024**, *14*, 1228. https://doi.org/10.3390/brainsci14121228.

3. Grasso, E.; Certo, F.; Ganau, M.; Bonomo, G.; Fiumanò, G.; Buscema, G.; Maugeri, A.; Agodi, A.; Barbagallo, G.M.V. Role of Virtual iMRI in Glioblastoma Surgery: Advantages, Limitations, and Correlation with iCT and Brain Shift. *Brain Sci.* **2025**, *15*, 35. https://doi.org/10.3390/brainsci15010035.
4. Guerrini, F.; Bertolino, L.; Safa, A.; Pittarello, M.; Parisi, A.; Beretta, L.V.; Zambelli, E.; Totis, F.; Campanaro, G.; Pavia, L.; et al. The Use of Technology-Based Simulation among Medical Students as a Global Innovative Solution for Training. *Brain Sci.* **2024**, *14*, 627. https://doi.org/10.3390/brainsci14070627
5. Alomari, A.A.; Eid, S.S.; Fraschetti, F.; Michelini, S.; Mastronardi, L. Comparative Analysis on Vestibular Schwannoma Surgery with and without Intraoperative Fluorescein Sodium Enhancement. *Brain Sci.* **2024**, *14*, 571. https://doi.org/10.3390/brainsci14060571.
6. Anselmi, L.; Anania, C.D.; Ubezio, M.C.; Farinaro, G.; Creatura, D.; Ortolina, A.; Tomei, M.; Baram, A.; Fornari, M. Cerebrospinal Fluid Leak Prevention in Intradural Spine Surgery: A Long Series Analysis of Closure with Non-Penetrating Titanium Clips. *Brain Sci.* **2024**, *14*, 1223. https://doi.org/10.3390/brainsci14121223.
7. Jee, T.K.; Yeon, J.Y.; Kim, K.H.; Kim, J.S.; Jeon, P. Flow Diversion for Cerebral Aneurysms: A Decade-Long Experience with Improved Outcomes and Predictors of Success. *Brain Sci.* **2024**, *14*, 847. https://doi.org/10.3390/brainsci14080847.
8. Khilar, S.; Dembinska-Kenner, A.; Hall, H.; Syrmos, N.; Ligarotti, G.K.; Plaha, P.; Apostolopoulos, V.; Chibbaro, S.; Barbagallo, G.M.V.; Ganau, M. Towards a New Dawn for Neuro-Oncology: Nanomedicine at the Service of Drug Delivery for Primary and Secondary Brain Tumours. *Brain Sci.* **2025**, *15*, 136. https://doi.org/10.3390/brainsci15020136.
9. Khan, S.; Kallis, L.; Mee, H.; El Hadwe, S.; Barone, D.; Hutchinson, P.; Kolias, A. Invasive Brain–Computer Interface for Communication: A Scoping Review. *Brain Sci.* **2025**, *15*, 336; https://doi.org/10.3390/brainsci15040336.

References

1. Kundu, M.; Ng, J.C.; Awuah, W.A.; Huang, H.; Yarlagadda, R.; Mehta, A.; Nansubuga, E.P.; Jiffry, R.; Abdul-Rahman, T.; Ou Yong, B.M.; et al. NeuroVerse: Neurosurgery in the era of Metaverse and other technological breakthroughs. *Postgrad. Med. J.* **2023**, *99*, 240–243. [CrossRef] [PubMed]
2. Yangi, K.; Hong, J.; Gholami, A.S.; On, T.J.; Reed, A.G.; Puppalla, P.; Chen, J.; Calderon Valero, C.E.; Xu, Y.; Li, B.; et al. Deep learning in neurosurgery: A systematic literature review with a structured analysis of applications across subspecialties. *Front. Neurol.* **2025**, *16*, 1532398. [CrossRef] [PubMed]
3. Cannizzaro, D.; Scalise, M.; Zancanella, C.; Paulli, S.; Peron, S.; Stefini, R. Comparative Evaluation of Major Robotic Systems in Microanastomosis Procedures: A Systematic Review of Current Capabilities and Future Potential. *Brain Sci.* **2024**, *14*, 1235. [CrossRef] [PubMed]
4. Wessel, K.J.; Dahmann, S.; Kueckelhaus, M. Expanding Applications and Future of Robotic Microsurgery. *J. Craniofac. Surg.* **2025**, *36*, 367–371. [CrossRef] [PubMed]
5. Reyes, J.S.; Lohia, V.N.; Almeida, T.; Niranjan, A.; Lunsford, L.D.; Hadjipanayis, C.G. Artificial intelligence in neurosurgery: A systematic review of applications, model comparisons, and ethical implications. *Neurosurg. Rev.* **2025**, *48*, 455. [CrossRef] [PubMed]
6. El-Hajj, V.G.; Gharios, M.; Edström, E.; Elmi-Terander, A. Artificial Intelligence in Neurosurgery: A Bibliometric Analysis. *World Neurosurg.* **2023**, *171*, 152–158.e4. [CrossRef] [PubMed]
7. Yilmaz, R.; Browd, S.; Donoho, D.A. Controversies in Artificial Intelligence in Neurosurgery. *Neurosurg. Clin. N. Am.* **2025**, *36*, 91–100. [CrossRef]

brain sciences

MDPI

Article

Role of Virtual iMRI in Glioblastoma Surgery: Advantages, Limitations, and Correlation with iCT and Brain Shift

Erica Grasso [1], Francesco Certo [1,2], Mario Ganau [3], Giulio Bonomo [1], Giuseppa Fiumanò [4], Giovanni Buscema [5], Andrea Maugeri [6], Antonella Agodi [6] and Giuseppe M. V. Barbagallo [1,2,*]

1 Department of Medical and Surgical Sciences and Advanced Technologies "G.F. Ingrassia", Neurological Surgery, Policlinico "G. Rodolico-San Marco" University Hospital, University of Catania, 95124 Catania, Italy; egrasso360@gmail.com (E.G.); cicciocerto@yahoo.it (F.C.); dott.giuliobonomo@gmail.com (G.B.)
2 Interdisciplinary Research Center on Brain Tumors Diagnosis and Treatment, University of Catania, 95124 Catania, Italy
3 Nuffield Department of Clinical Neurosciences, University of Oxford, Oxford OX1 2JD, UK; mario.ganau@alumni.harvard.edu
4 Department of Radiology and Radiotherapy, Policlinico "G. Rodolico-San Marco" University Hospital, University of Catania, 95124 Catania, Italy; gfiuman@sirm.org
5 Department of Anesthesia and Intensive Care, University Hospital Policlinico "G. Rodolico-San Marco", 95123 Catania, Italy; buscemagiovanni@gmail.com
6 Department of Medical and Surgical Sciences and Advanced Technologies "G.F. Ingrassia", University of Catania, 95124 Catania, Italy; andrea.maugeri@unict.it (A.M.); agodia@unict.it (A.A.)
* Correspondence: giuseppebarbagal@hotmail.com

Abstract: Background: Elastic image fusion (EIF) using an intraoperative CT (iCT) scan may enhance neuronavigation accuracy and compensate for brain shift. **Objective**: To evaluate the safety and reliability of the EIF algorithm (Virtual iMRI Cranial 4.5, Brainlab AG, Munich Germany, for the identification of residual tumour in glioblastoma surgery. Moreover, the impact of brain shift on software reliability is assessed. **Methods**: This ambispective study included 80 patients with a diagnosis of glioblastoma. Pre-operative MRI was elastically fused with an intraoperative CT scan (BodyTom; Samsung-Neurologica, Danvers, MA, USA) acquired at the end of the resection. Diagnostic specificity and the sensitivity of each tool was determined. The impact of brain shift on residual tumour was statistically analysed. An analysis of accuracy was performed through Target Registration Error (TRE) measurement after rigid image fusion (RIF) and EIF. A qualitative evaluation of each Virtual MRI image (VMRI) was performed. **Results**: VMRI identified residual tumour in 26/80 patients (32.5%), confirmed by post-operative MRI (true positive). Of these, 5 cases were left intentionally due to DES-positive responses, 8 cases underwent near maximal or subtotal resection, and 13 cases were not detected by iCT. However, in the other 27/80 cases (33.8%), VMRI reported residual tumour that was present neither on iCT nor on post-operative MRI (false positive). i-CT showed a sensitivity of 56% and specificity of 100%; VMRI demonstrated a sensitivity of 100% and specificity of 50%. Spearman correlation analysis showed a moderate correlation between pre-operative volume and VMRI tumour residual. Moreover, tumour involving insula or infiltrating more than one lobe displayed higher median values ($p = 0.023$) of virtual residual tumour. A statistically significant reduction towards lower TRE values after EIF was observed for test structures. **Conclusions**: Virtual iMRI was proven to be a feasible option to detect residual tumour. Its integration within a multimodal imaging protocol may provide neurosurgeons with intraoperatively updated imaging.

Keywords: brain shift; elastic image fusion; glioblastoma; intraoperative CT; rigid image fusion; Virtual iMRI; brain tumour surgery

1. Introduction

Brain shift represents a major source of inaccuracy in neuronavigation during the microsurgical removal of intracranial lesions [1–3]. Due to the heterogeneous nature of cerebral lesions [4] and the non-uniform distribution of brain shift [5,6], current rigid fusion (RIF) algorithms hardly deal with its complexity [7]. Indeed, linear fusion algorithms exclusively allow translations, rotations, scaling, and skewness to align datasets [8]. Recently, a novel tool for elastic image fusion (EIF), named Elements Virtual iMRI Cranial (Brainlab AG, Munich, Germany), has been developed to compensate for brain shift. Based on intraoperative imaging, this method elastically deforms pre-operative MRI data on intraoperative CT(iCT) imaging and updates the treatment plan [9]. To date, only a limited number of clinical studies have been reported using such a novel approach using either intraoperative MRI (iMR) [10–12] or the AIRO CT scanner [8,9,13–15]. Pilot studies reported significantly improved co-registration accuracy [8,10] and elastically updated DTI fibre tracts regarding intraoperative neuromonitoring and post-operative clinical status [11]. Conversely, the effectiveness of the EIF algorithm in visualising the residual tumour by elastically fusing intraoperative BodyTom CT images has not been explored yet.

Our work aimed to study two major aspects regarding the application of the algorithm in glioblastoma surgery. The first goal was to assess software accuracy to generate a "virtual" MRI and detect residual tumour compared to intraoperative CT images' sensitivity and specificity. Secondly, the impact of the major factors causing brain shift [2,7,16,17] was statistically analysed. Finally, image fusion accuracy was quantified by Target Registration Error (TRE) measurement and compared with previous data reported in the literature.

2. Materials and Methods

2.1. Patient Enrolment and Eligibility Criteria

In this cohort ambispective study, 80 patients with a diagnosis of glioblastoma (GBM, 2021 WHO classification) were included. Cases from January 2020 to August 2022 were analysed retrospectively, while the prospective cohort included patients from September 2022 to January 2024. Given the nature of this technological aid to surgical resection, the authors did not consider it ethically acceptable to perform a pure randomisation, and, rather, opted for a quasi-experimental cohort design, with retrospective analysis and prospective validation. Inclusion and exclusion criteria are reported in Table 1.

Table 1. Inclusion and exclusion criteria.

Inclusion Criteria	Exclusion Criteria
Diagnosis of glioblastoma	Different histological diagnosis
Supratentorial localisation	Infratentorial localisation
Neuroradiological dataset including pre- and post-operative MRI, intraoperative CT	Unavailable imaging dataset
Gross/Subtotal surgical excision	Surgical procedure different from gross/subtotal resection: biopsy, external ventricular drainage (DVE), ventriculoperitoneal shunt (DVP)

2.2. Data Acquisition and Volumetric Analysis

Data collection included the following information:

- Age
- Side and anatomical localisation of tumour within the brain
- Size of craniotomy

- Head position
- Ventricular opening
- Volumetric assessment:
  - Pre- and post-operative MRI tumour volume
  - Necrosis/tumour ratio (NTR)
  - Extent of resection (EOTR)
- Geometrical measurements for analysis of image accuracy:
  - Bifrontal ventricular width (referred to as "Evan's index" in the text)
  - Midline shift
  - Euclidean distance between anatomical landmarks after rigid image fusion (RIF) and elastic image fusion (EIF) algorithms.

Craniotomy was measured in the axial plane as the maximum distance between the external cortical bone edges. Patient positioning was classified as follows based on the angular tilt of head: 1: 0°, 2: 30°, 3: 45°, 4: 90°, 5: prone. Tumour location was classified as follows: group 1: tumours involving frontal lobe, group 2: tumours involving parietal lobe, group 3: tumours involving temporal lobe, group 4: tumours involving occipital lobe, group 5: tumours involving insula, group 6: tumours involving central core, group 7: tumours involving more than one lobe.

Volumes (expressed in cm^3) measured on pre-operative MRI included the following:

- "tumour": enhancing area on T1-weighted gadolinium (Gd)-enhanced sequence
- "necrosis": non-enhancing region within the tumour on T1-weighted Gd-enhanced MRI

Necrosis/ tumour ratio (NTR) was calculated as proposed by Henker et al. [18].

$$\mathrm{NTR} = \frac{\mathrm{NECROSIS}}{\mathrm{T_1 Vol}}$$

EOTR was then calculated using the Sanai and Berger [19] method and classified, according to the evidence-based recommendations proposed by Karschnia et al. [20], as 'biopsy', 'resection', 'subtotal resection', 'near total resection', 'complete resection', and 'supramaximal resection".

Virtual iMRI (VMRI) tumour residual was defined as the area not included in the resection cavity and refers to the total residual volume detected by the VMRI algorithm, encompassing both true positives and false positives. Quantitative volumetric measurements of these specific regions of interest (ROIs) were performed using a semi-automated contouring tool (Elements SmartBrush, Brainlab). All measurements were performed by the same researcher to rule out inter-observer variability. Additionally, measurements were double-checked in ten randomly selected cases by a researcher not involved in the original analysis to validate the results and assess inter-observer variability.

2.3. Intraoperative Multimodal Imaging Protocol

In all cases, an intraoperative multimodal imaging protocol previously described in [21,22] was applied; this included intraoperative CT (i-CT) (BodyTom; Samsung-Neurologica, Danvers, MA, USA), 5-Aminolevulinic acid (5-ALA) fluorescence, neuronavigation, and Intraoperative Neurophysiological Monitoring (IONM). Neuronavigation was conducted using a commercially available software (Cranial Navigation, Brainlab AG, Munich, Germany). The pre-operative dataset uploaded included at least a 3D T1-weighted gadolinium-enhancing MRI sequence. The first pre-operative post-contrast iCT was obtained after patient positioning to rigidly fuse it with the pre-operative MRI dataset. As resection was deemed to be complete, a second post-contrast iCT was acquired to estimate the extent of resection. If further resection proceeded due to evidence of residual tumour on iCT, a third post-contrast iCT was performed. At the end of surgical resection, VMRI was elastically fused to update the estimate extent of resection.

Quantitative evaluation of residual tumour was evaluated on post-operative T1-weighted gadolinium-enhancing MRI sequences acquired within 48 h.

2.4. Image Fusion Accuracy and Quantitation of the Target Registration Error

The spatial alignment of fused pre-operative and Virtual iMRI (VMRI) was assessed via Target Registration Error (TRE) measurements, which requires calculating Euclidean distance between manually defined landmarks [8,23–27]. In our study, the TREs between pre-operative MRI and iCT (after RIF) and between Virtual iMRI and iCT (after EIF), were measured as Euclidean distance between paired landmarks (Figure 1). Anterior–posterior and latero-lateral reference points were considered in our measurements and included the following anatomical structures:

- Maximum cortical displacement in lateral and cranio-caudal directions;
- Anterior communicating artery at its junction with A1 segment (AComm);
- Basilar apex;
- Midline shift;
- Evan's index.

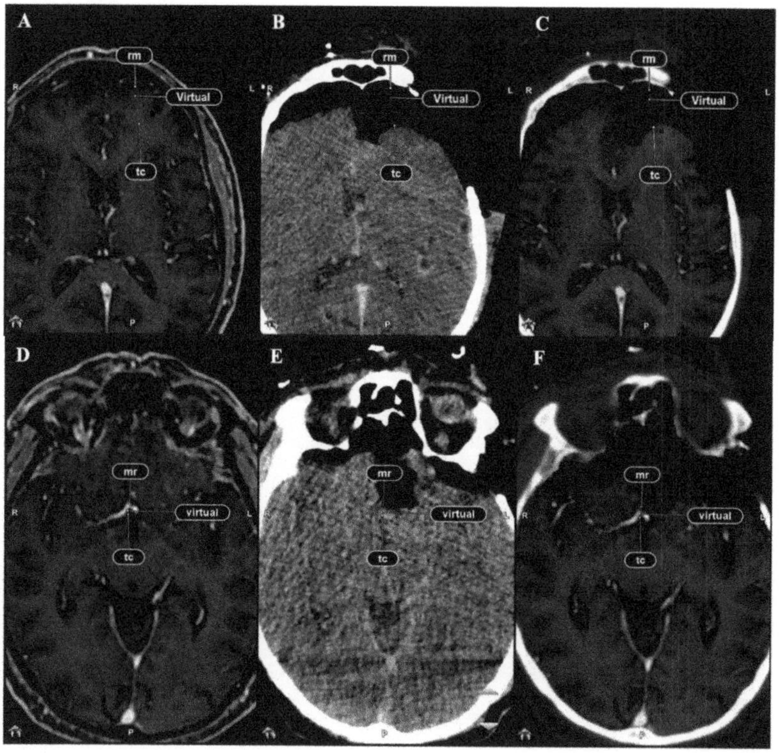

Figure 1. Identification of corresponding anatomic landmarks used for TRE calculation after RIF and EIF. (**A**) Pre-operative MRI with corresponding cortical points. (**B**) iCT scan image with corresponding cortical point. (**C**) Virtual iMRI with corresponding cortical points. (**D**) Pre-operative MRI with AComm set as reference point. (**E**) iCT scan image with corresponding AComm. (**F**) Virtual iMRI with corresponding AComm.

Anterior communicating artery (AComm) and Basilar apex were considered control structures, while cortical shift, midline shift, and Evan's index were the test structures considered as parameters of cortical, parenchymal, and ventricular deformation, respectively. To better quantify the effect of brain shift on ventricular structures, in the statistical analysis, only the maximum bifrontal width of ventricles based on previous Evan's index was considered.

2.5. Qualitative Comparison of iCT, Virtual iMRI, and Post-Operative MRI

Two expert neurosurgeons reviewed six different parameters resulting from EIF using a side-by-side approach (Figure 2). The observers primarily compared the VMRI images to the iCT data and, secondarily, VMRI and post-operative MRI. More specifically, factors analysed in the comparison between i-CT and Virtual iMRI were matching of relevant anatomical structures, residual tumour on i-CT, and matching of residual tumour on both images. Similarly, the analysis between VMRI and post-operative MR included matching of residual tumour, matching of surgical cavity edges, and overall quality of virtual image.

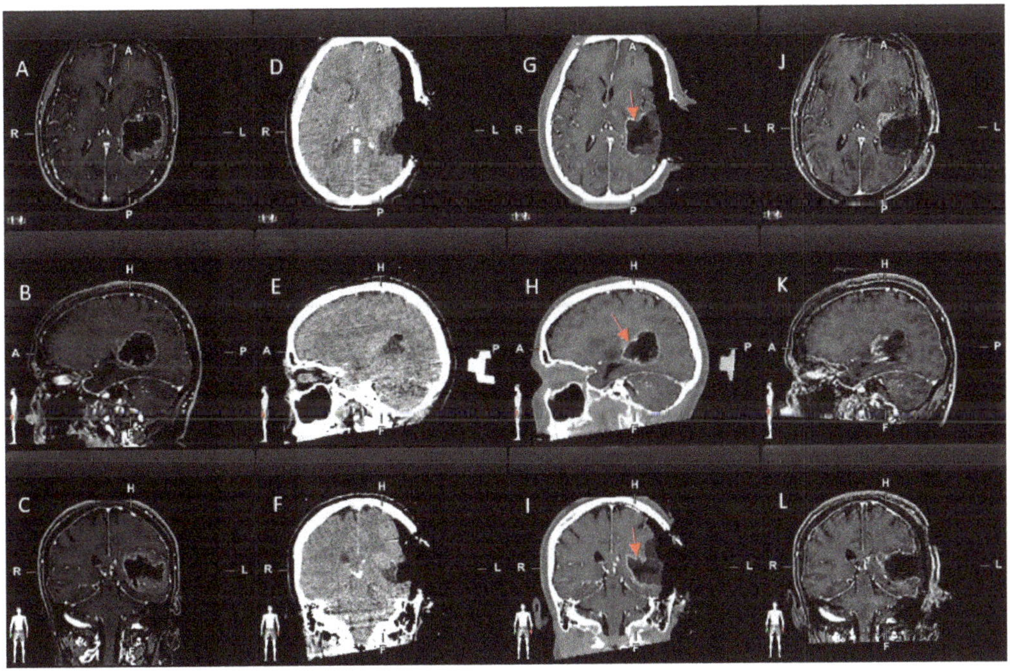

Figure 2. Method adopted for assessing the accuracy of Virtual iMRI. (**A–C**) Pre-operative MRI in axial, sagittal, and coronal view. (**D–F**) Post-contrast i-CT scan in axial, sagittal, and coronal view. (**G–I**) Virtual iMRI image with axial, sagittal, and coronal view. (**J–L**) Post-operative MRI in axial, sagittal, and coronal view. Red arrows indicate residual tumour on Virtual iMRI which is not included in the resection cavity (grey area).

Accuracy was rated on a scale ranging from 1 to 5: 1, matching < 10 slices in at least 2 projections; 2, matching between 10 and 20 slices in at least 2 projections; 3, matching between 10 and 20 slices in the 3 projections; 4, matching > 20 slices in the 3 projections; 5, complete matching. Overall quality was rated as 1, low quality; 2, low-medium quality; 3, intermediate; 4, medium-high quality; 5, high quality.

2.6. Statistical Analysis

Data analysis was conducted using SPSS (version 29.0; IBM). The normality of the data and the suitability for parametric tests were assessed using the Shapiro–Wilk test. Descriptive statistics summarised quantitative variables using mean and standard error or median and interquartile range (IQR) based on their distribution (Table 2).

Table 2. Summarised quantitative variables expressed as mean and standard deviation (SD) or median and interquartile range (IQR) based on their distribution. Legend: NTR: necrosis/tumour ratio; EOTR: extent of resection.

VARIABLE	Frequency, Mean (SD), or Median (IQR) n = 80 Patients
Male	44
Female	36
Mean age (years)	61 years
Median craniotomy size (mm)	70 (21.5)
Head positioning	
0°	9
30°	16
45°	17
90°	21
Prone	12
Tumour location	
Frontal lobe	22
Parietal lobe	10
Temporal lobe	18
Occipital lobe	3
Insula	12
Central core	4
Median tumour volume on pre-operative Gd-enhanced MRI (cm^3)	33.5 (33.9)
Median necrosis volume (cm^3)	10 (20.4)
Median NTR (with 0 meaning that tumour was entirely fleshy and 1 fully necrotic or colloid)	0.37 (0.44)
Median tumour residual volume on Virtual iMRI (cm^3)	1.88 (7.7)
Median tumour volume on post-operative Gd-enhanced MRI (cm^3)	0 (0.8)
Mean EOTR	97%

Spearman correlation analysis explored relationships among seven phenomena (residual tumour after EIF, lateral and cranio-caudal cortical shift, midline shift variation, Evan's index variation, Basilar apex shift, AComm shift) and three parameters (craniotomy, tumour volume measured on pre-operative T1 gadolinium-enhancing MRI sequences, and NTR). Correlations were expressed as Spearman rho coefficients and associated p-values. Correlation strength was categorised according to Critical Values for Spearman's Rank

Order Correlation. Differences in the seven phenomena, categorised by ventricular opening, tumour localisation, and patient positioning, were analysed using either the Mann–Whitney or Kruskal–Wallis test.

Unadjusted linear regression models evaluated parameters potentially associated with residual tumour after EIF, with craniotomy, pre-operative T1, gadolinium enhancing, tumour volume, NTR, ventricular opening, tumour location, and patient positioning as independent variables. Adjusted linear regression analysis was applied for variables exhibiting significant associations in unadjusted models. β coefficients along with their standard error (SE) quantified the strength and direction of associations, and the coefficient of determination (R^2) assessed the proportion of variance explained by independent variables. Comparison of lateral and cranio-caudal shift, anterior communicating artery, Basilar apex, Evan's index, and midline shift after rigid and elastic fusion, as well as TRE quantities, was conducted using the Wilcoxon signed-rank test for paired samples. Due to the exploratory nature of the analyses, aiming to identify potential trends and associations rather than confirmatory testing, adjustments for multiple comparisons were not applied. A significance level of 0.05 and, if necessary, a 95% confidence interval, were applied to all analyses.

3. Results

3.1. Residual Tumour

Residual tumour was detected on post-operative MRI in 26 out of 80 patients (32.5%). Among these, intraoperative CT (iCT) correctly identified residual tumour in 17 patients (21.2%) and led to further resection in 12 cases, resulting in complete (4), near-complete (4), and subtotal (4) resections. In the other five cases, further resection could not be performed because the lesion was located in eloquent brain areas, or it showed positive responses to direct electrical stimulation (DES). In the remaining 13 out of 80 cases (16.3%), iCT failed to detect the residual tumour (false negative). No false positives were observed. Therefore, iCT showed 56% sensitivity and 100% specificity.

By contrast, VMRI identified residual tumour in 26/80 patients (32.5%), further confirmed by post-operative MRI (true positive). Of these, 5 cases were left intentionally due to DES-positive responses, 8 cases underwent near maximal or subtotal resection, and 13 cases were not detected in the iCT. However, in the other 27/80 cases (33.8%), VMRI reported residual tumour that was present neither on iCT nor on post-operative MRI (false positive). No false negatives were observed. Considering these results, Virtual iMRI demonstrated 100% sensitivity and 50% specificity (Table 3).

Table 3. Confusion matrix reporting the FP: false positive; FN: false negative; TP: true positive; TN: true negative; PPV: positive predictive value; NPV: negative predictive value of iCT and Virtual iMRI. These data were utilised to calculate the diagnostic sensitivity and specificity of each imaging tool.

	TC	Virtual iMRI
FP	0	27
FN	13	0
TP	17	26
TN	50	27
SENSITIVITY	0.56	1
SPECIFICITY	1	0.5
PPV	1	0.49
NPV	0.79	1

Figures 3 and 4 depict the results of bivariate analyses for all parameters under examination.

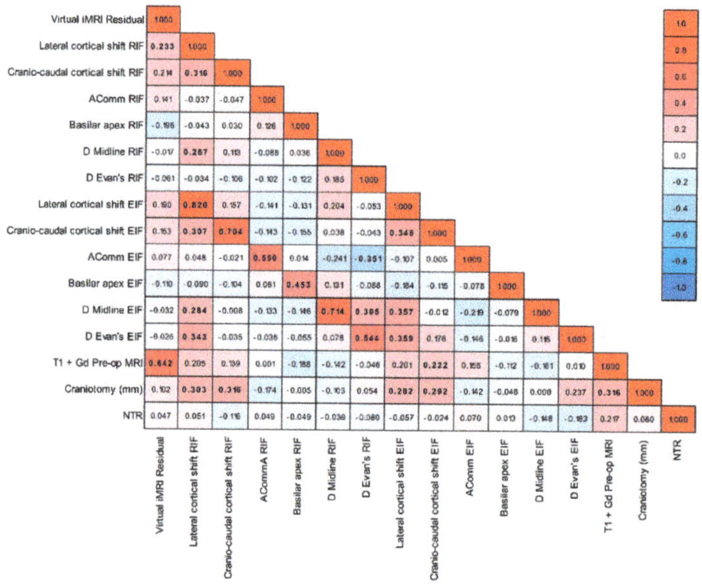

Figure 3. Heatmap illustrating the correlations among the quantitative variables under investigation. The figure presents Spearman correlation coefficients ranging from −1 (depicted in blue) to +1 (depicted in red). Correlations that are statistically significant (p-values < 0.05) are highlighted in bold.

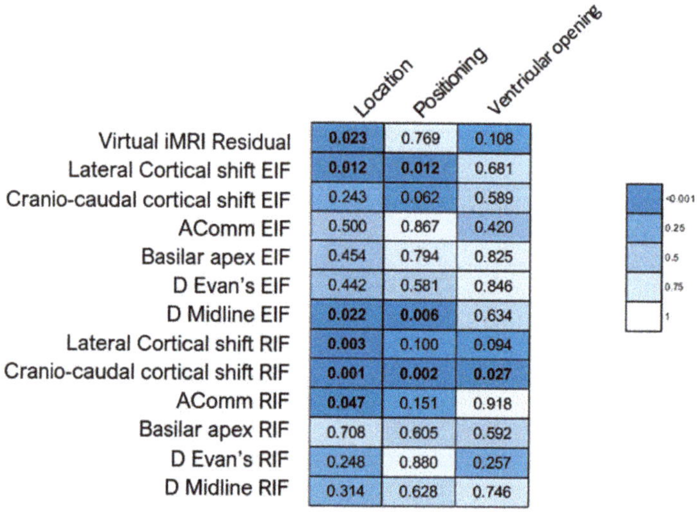

Figure 4. Heatmap illustrating the differences among the quantitative variables according to tumour location, patient positioning, and ventricular opening. The figure displays the p-values obtained through Mann–Whitney or Kruskal–Wallis tests. Statistically significant p-values (<0.05) are highlighted in bold.

A moderate positive correlation was observed between VMRI tumour residual and pre-operative gadolinium-enhanced MRI (rho = 0.642; $p < 0.001$). The β coefficient from the simple linear regression suggests that, with each one-unit increase in pre-operative gadolinium-enhanced MRI, the VMRI tumour residual is expected to increase by 0.131 units. The R2 value of 0.327 suggests that approximately 32.7% of the variability in the dependent variable is explained by the independent variable in the model (Figure 5A). This means that the model accounts for a moderate proportion of the total variability in the dependent variable. Conversely, craniotomy and NTR showed non-significant correlations (rho = 0.102, p = 0.370 and rho= 0.047, p = 0.682, respectively). The absence of a linear relationship is corroborated by the scatter plots depicted in Figure 5B,C.

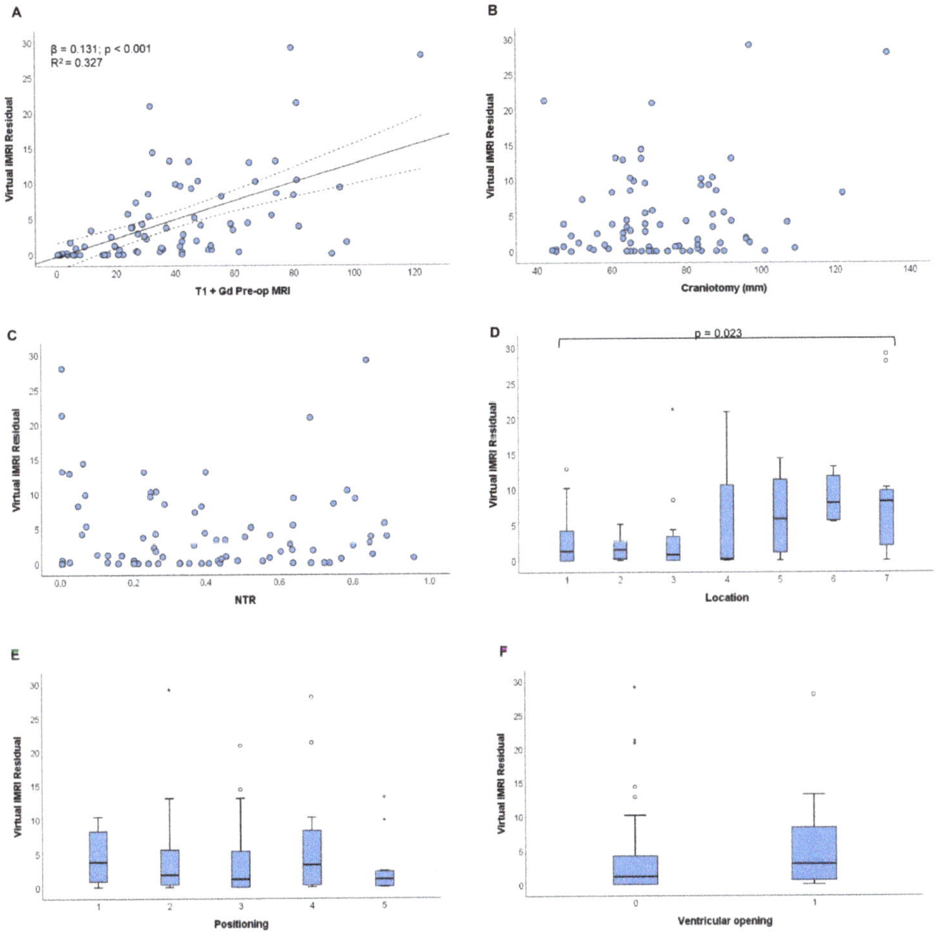

Figure 5. Factors potentially associated with residual tumour on Virtual iMRI. Scatter plots in Figures (**A–C**) show the relationship of Virtual iMRI residual with pre-operative T1 + Gd tumour volume, craniotomy, and NTR; in Figure (**A**), the solid line and dashed lines represent the linear regression line and its confidence intervals, respectively, for the statistically significant relationship between Virtual iMRI residual and pre-operative T1 + Gd tumour volume. Box plots in Figures (**D–F**) illustrate the variations in Virtual iMRI residual based on tumour location, patient positioning, and ventricular opening; the p-value in Figure (**D**) is determined by the Kruskal–Wallis test.

Variations in VMRI tumour residual were observable across various tumour locations (p = 0.023), particularly displaying higher median values within groups 5–7 (Figure 5D). No significant differences in VMRI residual were observed concerning head position (p = 0.769) and ventricular opening (p = 0.108) (Figure 5E,F).

The results from the adjusted linear regression model confirm the association between pre-operative gadolinium-enhanced MRI and tumour location with Virtual iMRI residual. More precisely, the VMRI residual increases by 0.120 units for each one-unit increment in pre-operative gadolinium-enhanced MRI ($\beta = 0.120$; SE = 0.020; $p < 0.001$). Furthermore, individuals belonging to tumour location groups 5–7 demonstrate higher values compared to those in other groups ($\beta = 3.710$; SE = 1.165; $p = 0.002$). The R2 increased compared to the unadjusted model, indicating that approximately 40.5% of the variability in the dependent variable is explained by the adjusted model.

3.2. *Analysis on Accuracy: Quantitation of the Target Registration Error*

For descriptive purposes, mean TRE values of paired anatomical landmarks measured between pre-operative MRI and iCT (after RIF) and between Virtual iMRI and iCT (after EIF) are summarised in Table 4.

Table 4. Target Registration Error (TRE) values reported between pre-operative MRI and iCT (after RIF) and between Virtual iMRI and iCT (after EIF) of paired anatomical landmarks. Note that Evan's index refers to bifrontal ventricular diameter.

	Maximum		Minimum		Mean ± SD	
	RIF	**EIF**	**RIF**	**EIF**	**RIF**	**EIF**
Lateral cortical shift	32	22	0	0	12.5 ± 8.9	9.6 ± 6.8
Cranio-caudal cortical shift	30	22	0	0	10.9 ± 7.7	7.8 ± 5.6
Anterior communicating artery	3	5	−5	−4	−0.8 ± 1.6	−0.1 ± 1.4
Basilar apex	2	2	−2	−3	−0.3 ± 0.8	−0.1 ± 0.8
D Midline shift	9	7	−4	−6	1.5 ± 3	1 ± 2.6
D Evan's index	19	11	−3	−10	4.8 ± 4.5	2.1 ± 3.8

Figure 6 shows the comparison of lateral and cranio-caudal shift, anterior communicating artery, Basilar apex, Evan's index, and midline shift after rigid and elastic fusion. Compared to post-RIF evaluation, significantly lower values after EIF were evident for lateral and cranio-caudal shift ($p = 0.001$ and $p < 0.001$, respectively), Evan's index ($p < 0.001$), and midline shift ($p = 0.008$). Conversely, no significant reduction was observed for control structures (AComm and Basilar apex) after EIF ($p = 0.169$ and $p = 0.218$, respectively).

Concerning lateral and cranio-caudal cortical shift, certain correlations and differences were observed. While lateral cortical shift displayed weak correlations with craniotomy (rho = 0.282; $p = 0.012$), cranio-caudal cortical shift demonstrated weak correlations with both T1-enhanced MRI (rho = 0.222; $p = 0.049$) and craniotomy (rho = 0.292; $p = 0.009$). The lateral cortical shift also varied based on tumour location and positioning (p-values = 0.012), indicating significant pairwise differences between groups 1 and 5 of tumour location ($p = 0.007$) and groups 4 and 5 of positioning ($p = 0.029$). Comparable findings emerged when assessing the values after RIF, revealing moderate correlations between craniotomy and both lateral and cranio-caudal cortical shift, along with significant differences by tumour location, positioning, and ventricular opening (Figures 3 and 4). Midline shift also exhibited differences based on tumour location and positioning ($p = 0.022$ and $0 = 0.006$, respectively; Figure 3). Specifically, significant differences were observed between groups 1 and 5 for location ($p = 0.049$) and between pairs 1–4 and 2–4 for positioning ($p = 0.007$ and $p = 0.046$, respectively).

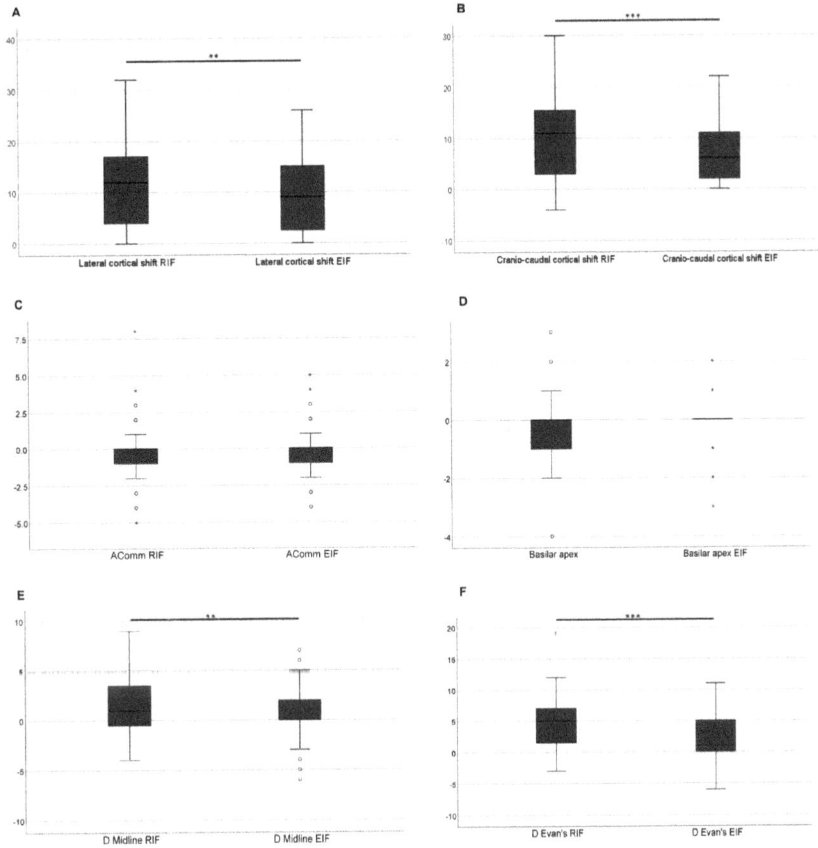

Figure 6. Comparison of lateral (**A**) and cranio-caudal shift (**B**), anterior communicating artery (**C**), Basilar apex (**D**), midline shift (**E**), and Evan's index (**F**) after rigid and elastic fusion. Statistical significance is denoted as ** for p-value < 0.01, and *** for p-value < 0.001, based on the Wilcoxon signed-rank test for paired samples.

3.3. Qualitative Evaluation

On average, the matching of relevant anatomical structures between VMRI data and iCT scan resulted in score of 3.5 and approximately 3.3 regarding the matching of residual tumour. Similarly, the analysis between VMRI and post-operative MRI concerning the matching of residual tumour and the matching of surgical cavity edges showed a mean score of 3.2 and 3.3, respectively. Overall, quality image yielded a mean score of 3.4 meaning that, on average, VMRI accuracy was rated as intermediate. The evaluation performed in ten randomly selected cases was double-checked by a researcher not involved in the original analysis, which confirmed the absence of significant inter-observer variability in the qualitative evaluation of images.

4. Discussion

We described the use of a novel EIF algorithm to detect residual tumour and to update intraoperative neuronavigation. Unlike RIF algorithms, this tool deforms the preoperative plan, taking into account several physical forces such as gravity, cerebrospinal-fluid-related force, and the modelling of the collision of FEM-voxels, both with other soft- or stiff-tissue-related FEM-Voxels and with the rigid skull [8].

Compared to the few studies in the literature, ours provides new insights for different reasons. In previous studies, either iMR [10–12] or the AIRO CT scanner [8,9,13–15] were used. To the best of our knowledge, this is the first study reporting the results of intraoperative BodyTom CT images elastically fused using Virtual iMRI.

We have illustrated the diagnostic sensitivity and specificity of these two techniques (BodyTom i-CT and Virtual iMRI) in visualising residual tumour. As reported above, iCT showed 56% sensitivity and 100% specificity. Conversely, Virtual iMRI demonstrated 100% sensitivity and 50% specificity. These results suggest that the integration of this novel algorithm into the intraoperative workflow can offer the possibility of combining maximal iCT specificity with the higher sensitivity of EIF algorithm. Recently, Mazzucchi et al. [13] reported a sensitivity of 1 and a specificity of 0.33 of Virtual iMRI in glioblastoma surgery. However, the heterogeneity of the cohort, with only nine glioblastoma cases, and the absence of any analysis on the causes of false positives prevent us from comparing results. Conversely, we analysed the known factors causing brain shift to elucidate potential explanations for the large number of false positives. The results obtained from the adjusted linear regression model showed that EIF algorithm tends to report higher "virtual" residual tumour, which is quantitatively influenced mainly by the pre-operative volume and by tumour location, with tumour involving insula or infiltrating more than one lobe carrying the major brain shift effects. These results led us to hypothesise that smaller virtual residual tumours might be caused by errors occurring in the semi-automatic registration phase, whereas, in bigger tumours, the algorithm failed to include tumour into the resection cavity due to the major influence of brain shift. Compared to our study, Nimsky et al. [7] also documented the role of craniotomy size, resection volume, patient position, and tissue characteristics on brain shift after RIF using iMRI. As already stated by Hartkens et al. [28], we agree that the combination of these factors, rather than their isolated contribution, eventually determines the final result. Further studies with a larger cohort of patients will be needed to better assess how the interplay between these factors causes the EIF algorithm to crash.

Considering our results, surgeons should be cautious in planning the further resection of any eventual "virtual" residual tumour, especially when an increased risk of "false positive" virtual residual tumour can be suspected (i.e., high pre-operative tumour volume, insula or multiple lobe infiltration). In such cases, resorting to other intraoperative tools might settle the doubts between a "false positive" and a "true positive" residual. Several additional devices might help the surgeon. In 2014, Stummer et al. [29] demonstrated that 5-ALA fluorescence predicted solid and infiltrating tumour and concluded that fluorescence appears superior to contrast enhancement on MRI for indicating residual tumour. More recently, Roder et al. [30], in a nonrandomised prospective controlled trial (PCT), demonstrated the non-superiority of iMRI compared to 5-ALA, which might be advantageous economically and timing-wise given the significantly longer operating room times of iMRI. Intraoperative ultrasound (iUS) has been widely accepted as a real-time image-guided tool for the excision of intracranial lesions [3,30–32]. Moreover, in 2020, Della Pepa et al. [33] achieved the best results in terms of the extent of resection through a combination of both techniques, where the 5-ALA-guided procedure is followed by a final survey with iUS. In our institutional experience, the multimodal intraoperative imaging protocol based on the combination of intraoperative Ultrasound (iUS), intraoperative Computed Tomography (i-CT) integrated with 5-ALA fluorescence, and neuromonitoring-guided resection proved to safely increase the extent of resection [21,34]. We assume that, while the EIF algorithm might unveil residual tumour not clearly recognisable on the iCT, its confirmation should be achieved with the available intraoperative tools, especially in those cases in which a major influence of brain shift is suspected.

Regardless of tumour volume and location, the drawing of the resection cavity, as well as iCT image quality, appeared to be key. In terms of overall image quality, indeed, the worst results were observed when key anatomical structures (i.e., ventricles) were hardly distinguishable and the surgical cavity collapsed due to several factors (re-expansion of the surrounding parenchyma, gravity, etc.). In these cases, indeed, the manual drawing of the resection cavity might be challenging, and inaccuracies in tumour boundary delineation result in a "false positive" residual tumour. Autonomous drawing based on generative artificial intelligence, or a standardised step-by-step drawing protocol will be needed to address this problem and improve the software's reliability.

Finally, regarding the analysis of navigation reliability, the registration of accuracy performed via the landmark-based measurements of the Target Registration Error after RIF and EIF revealed no significant change in control structures. Conversely, a statistically significant reduction towards lower TRE values was observed for lateral and cranio-caudal shift, Evan's index, and midline shift. Our results are in line with those presented by Riva et al. [8] and Mazzucchi et al. [10], who reported reduced TRE values after EIF, with no significant change in TRE measurements for control structures as well. Overall, the elastic fusion algorithm proved to increase navigation accuracy by reducing the deformation occurring in both the parenchyma and ventricular system compared to standard rigid fusion algorithms [35].

Limitations and Future Directions

This work has some limitations. First, the limited amount of data might have weakened the strength of the statistical analysis. Larger studies with the integration of multi centre data are needed to provide surgeons with an effective and validated tool to manage a highly complex phenomenon like brain shift. A great bias is the consequence of measuring fusion accuracy by determining the TRE, which is dependent on iCT interpretation.

Similarly, as drawing the resection cavity to perform Virtual iMRI is operator-dependent, the software still lacks a standardised step-by-step drawing protocol, which may limit its reproducibility. Autonomous drawing based on generative artificial intelligence could, in the future, address this problem. Additionally, the availability of new CT devices with a software that reduces metal artifacts and noise might increase the iCT image quality, leading to the easier drawing of surgical cavity and elastic fusion itself. Nonetheless, such a leap forward is still long to come because, at present, applications in image interpretation are lagging behind compared to text analysis.

5. Conclusions

This study reports our early experience in the clinical feasibility, safety, and reliability of a novel EIF algorithm (Virtual iMRI, Brainlab) and proposes a new approach for the intraoperative evaluation of residual tumour in glioblastoma surgery. It also sheds light on factors which influence the "virtual" image. The algorithm proved to globally enhance the spatial image fusion, increasing neuronavigation accuracy.

Author Contributions: Each author has made substantial contributions, has approved the submitted version, and agrees to be personally accountable for the author's own contributions and for ensuring that questions related to the accuracy or integrity of any part of the work, even ones in which the author was not personally involved, are appropriately investigated, resolved, and documented in the literature. Conceptualisation, E.G., F.C. and G.M.V.B.; Methodology, E.G. and F.C.; Software, F.C. and G.M.V.B.; Validation, E.G., F.C. and G.B. (Giulio Bonomo); Formal Analysis, A.M. and A.A.; Investigation, E.G. and F.C.; Resources, G.F. and G.M.V.B.; Data Curation, E.G., A.M. and A.A.; Writing—Original Draft Preparation, E.G. and F.C.; Writing—Review and Editing, F.C., M.G. and

G.M.V.B.; Visualisation, G.B. (Giovanni Buscema)., M.G. and G.M.V.B.; Supervision, F.C. and G.M.V.B. All authors have read and agreed to the published version of the manuscript.

Funding: This research received no external funding.

Institutional Review Board Statement: Not applicable. Neither Institutional Review Board approval nor specific patient consent were required as the study did not change or influence the standard of care usually provided in our institution to patients suffering from brain glioblastoma. Our study focused on a novel intraoperative image analysis (Virtual MRI) performed using a new software, but did not lead to surgical strategy changes.

Informed Consent Statement: Not applicable.

Data Availability Statement: The data presented in this study are available upon request from the corresponding author due to privacy concerns.

Acknowledgments: We are grateful to the Department of Medical and Surgical Sciences and Advanced Technologies "G.F. Ingrassia", University of Catania, Italy, for the financial support for publication.

Conflicts of Interest: The authors have no personal, financial, or institutional interest in any of the drugs, materials, or devices described in this article.

References

1. Reinges, M.H.T.; Nguyen, H.-H.; Krings, T.; Hütter, B.-O.; Rohde, V.; Gilsbach, J.M. Course of Brain Shift during Microsurgical Resection of Supratentorial Cerebral Lesions: Limits of Conventional Neuronavigation. *Acta Neurochir.* **2004**, *146*, 369–377. [CrossRef] [PubMed]
2. Gerard, I.J.; Kersten-Oertel, M.; Petrecca, K.; Sirhan, D.; Hall, J.A.; Collins, D.L. Brain Shift in Neuronavigation of Brain Tumors: A Review. *Med. Image Anal.* **2017**, *35*, 403–420. [CrossRef] [PubMed]
3. Ganau, M.; Ligarotti, G.K.; Apostolopoulos, V. Real-Time Intraoperative Ultrasound in Brain Surgery: Neuronavigation and Use of Contrast-Enhanced Image Fusion. *Quant. Imaging Med. Surg.* **2019**, *9*, 35058–35358. [CrossRef]
4. Ohue, S.; Kumon, Y.; Nagato, S.; Kohno, S.; Harada, H.; Nakagawa, K.; Kikuchi, K.; Miki, H.; Ohnishi, T. Evaluation of Intraoperative Brain Shift Using an Ultrasound-Linked Navigation System for Brain Tumor Surgery. *Neurol. Med. Chir.* **2010**, *50*, 291–300. [CrossRef] [PubMed]
5. Becker, S.; Mang, A.; Toma, A.; Buzug, T.M. In-Silico Oncology: An Approximate Model of Brain Tumor Mass Effect Based on Directly Manipulated Free Form Deformation. *Int. J. CARS* **2010**, *5*, 607–622. [CrossRef] [PubMed]
6. Nabavi, A.; Gering, D.T.; Mehta, V.; Ferrant, M.; Hata, N.; Schwartz, R.B.; Iii, W.M.W.; Jolesz, F.A. Serial Intraoperative Magnetic Resonance Imaging of Brain Shift. *Neurosurgery* **2001**, *48*, 787–798. [PubMed]
7. Nimsky, C.; Ganslandt, O.; Cerny, S.; Hastreiter, P.; Greiner, G.; Fahlbusch, R. Quantification of, Visualization of, and Compensation for Brain Shift Using Intraoperative Magnetic Resonance Imaging. *Neurosurgery* **2000**, *47*, 1070–1080. [CrossRef]
8. Riva, M.; Hiepe, P.; Frommert, M.; Divenuto, I.; Gay, L.G.; Sciortino, T.; Nibali, M.C.; Rossi, M.; Pessina, F.; Bello, L. Intraoperative Computed Tomography and Finite Element Modelling for Multimodal Image Fusion in Brain Surgery. *Oper. Surg.* **2020**, *18*, 531–541. [CrossRef]
9. Mazzucchi, E.; La Rocca, G.; Hiepe, P.; Pignotti, F.; Galieri, G.; Policicchio, D.; Boccaletti, R.; Rinaldi, P.; Gaudino, S.; Ius, T.; et al. Intraoperative Integration of Multimodal Imaging to Improve Neuronavigation: A Technical Note. *World Neurosurg.* **2022**, *164*, 330–340. [CrossRef] [PubMed]
10. Negwer, C.; Hiepe, P.; Meyer, B.; Krieg, S.M. Elastic Fusion Enables Fusion of Intraoperative Magnetic Resonance Imaging Data with Preoperative Neuronavigation Data. *World Neurosurg.* **2020**, *142*, e223–e228. [CrossRef]
11. Ille, S.; Schroeder, A.; Wagner, A.; Negwer, C.; Kreiser, K.; Meyer, B.; Krieg, S.M. Intraoperative MRI–Based Elastic Fusion for Anatomically Accurate Tractography of the Corticospinal Tract: Correlation with Intraoperative Neuromonitoring and Clinical Status. *Neurosurg. Focus* **2021**, *50*, E9. [CrossRef]
12. Zhang, W.; Ille, S.; Schwendner, M.; Wiestler, B.; Meyer, B.; Krieg, S.M. Tracking Motor and Language Eloquent White Matter Pathways with Intraoperative Fiber Tracking versus Preoperative Tractography Adjusted by Intraoperative MRI–Based Elastic Fusion. *J. Neurosurg.* **2022**, *137*, 1114–1123. [CrossRef]

13. Mazzucchi, E.; Cavlak, L.B.; Pignotti, F.; La Rocca, G.; Cusumano, D.; Rinaldi, P.; Olivi, A.; Sabatino, G. Evaluation of the Extent of Resection of Intracranial Tumors with Virtual Intraoperative MRI: A Case Series. *J. Neurosurg.* **2024**, *141*, 695–701. [CrossRef]
14. Kim, J.T.; Di, L.; Etame, A.B.; Olson, S.; Vogelbaum, M.A.; Tran, N.D. Use of Virtual Magnetic Resonance Imaging to Compensate for Brain Shift during Image-Guided Surgery: Illustrative Case. *J. Neurosurg. Case Lessons* **2022**, *3*, CASE21683. [CrossRef]
15. Senova, S.; Lefaucheur, J.-P.; Brugières, P.; Ayache, S.S.; Tazi, S.; Bapst, B.; Abhay, K.; Langeron, O.; Edakawa, K.; Palfi, S.; et al. Case Report: Multimodal Functional and Structural Evaluation Combining Pre-Operative nTMS Mapping and Neuroimaging With Intraoperative CT-Scan and Brain Shift Correction for Brain Tumor Surgical Resection. *Front. Hum. Neurosci.* **2021**, *15*, 646268. [CrossRef] [PubMed]
16. Schnaudigel, S.; Preul, C.; Ugur, T.; Mentzel, H.J.; Witte, O.W.; Tittgemeyer, M.; Hagemann, G. Positional Brain Deformation Visualized With Magnetic Resonance Morphometry. *Neurosurgery* **2010**, *66*, 376. [CrossRef]
17. Trantakis, C.; Tittgemeyer, M.; Schneider, J.-P.; Lindner, D.; Winkler, D.; Strauß, G.; Meixensberger, J. Investigation of Time-Dependency of Intracranial Brain Shift and Its Relation to the Extent of Tumor Removal Using Intra-Operative MRI. *Neurol. Res.* **2003**, *25*, 9–12. [CrossRef]
18. Henker, C.; Kriesen, T.; Glass, Ä.; Schneider, B.; Piek, J. Volumetric Quantification of Glioblastoma: Experiences with Different Measurement Techniques and Impact on Survival. *J. Neurooncol.* **2017**, *135*, 391–402. [CrossRef] [PubMed]
19. Sanai, N.; Berger, M.S. Glioma extent of resection and its impact on patient outcome. *Neurosurgery* **2008**, *62*, 753–766. [CrossRef]
20. Karschnia, P.; Vogelbaum, M.A.; van den Bent, M.; Cahill, D.P.; Bello, L.; Narita, Y.; Berger, M.S.; Weller, M.; Tonn, J.-C. Evidence-Based Recommendations on Categories for Extent of Resection in Diffuse Glioma. *Eur. J. Cancer* **2021**, *149*, 23–33. [CrossRef]
21. Vincenzo Barbagallo, G.M.; Certo, F.; Di Gregorio, S.; Maione, M.; Garozzo, M.; Peschillo, S.; Altieri, R. Recurrent High-Grade Glioma Surgery: A Multimodal Intraoperative Protocol to Safely Increase Extent of Tumor Resection and Analysis of Its Impact on Patient Outcome. *Neurosurg. Focus* **2021**, *50*, E20. [CrossRef] [PubMed]
22. Certo, F.; Altieri, R.; Grasso, G.; Barbagallo, G.M.V. Role of I-CT, i-US, and Neuromonitoring in Surgical Management of Brain Cavernous Malformations and Arteriovenous Malformations: A Case Series. *World Neurosurg.* **2022**, *159*, 402–408. [CrossRef] [PubMed]
23. Xiao, Y.; Rivaz, H.; Chabanas, M.; Fortin, M.; Machado, I.; Ou, Y.; Heinrich, M.P.; Schnabel, J.A.; Zhong, X.; Maier, A.; et al. Evaluation of MRI to Ultrasound Registration Methods for Brain Shift Correction: The CuRIOUS2018 Challenge. *IEEE Trans. Med. Imaging* **2020**, *39*, 777–786. [CrossRef] [PubMed]
24. Machado, I.; Toews, M.; George, E.; Unadkat, P.; Essayed, W.; Luo, J.; Teodoro, P.; Carvalho, H.; Martins, J.; Golland, P.; et al. Deformable MRI-Ultrasound Registration Using Correlation-Based Attribute Matching for Brain Shift Correction: Accuracy and Generality in Multi-Site Data. *Neuroimage* **2019**, *202*, 116094. [CrossRef]
25. Furuse, M.; Ikeda, N.; Kawabata, S.; Park, Y.; Takeuchi, K.; Fukumura, M.; Tsuji, Y.; Kimura, S.; Kanemitsu, T.; Yagi, R.; et al. Influence of Surgical Position and Registration Methods on Clinical Accuracy of Navigation Systems in Brain Tumor Surgery. *Sci. Rep.* **2023**, *13*, 2644. [CrossRef] [PubMed]
26. Mazzucchi, E.; Hiepe, P.; Langhof, M.; La Rocca, G.; Pignotti, F.; Rinaldi, P.; Sabatino, G. Automatic Rigid Image Fusion of Preoperative MR and Intraoperative US Acquired after Craniotomy. *Cancer Imaging* **2023**, *23*, 37. [CrossRef]
27. Wang, M.N.; Song, Z.J. Properties of the Target Registration Error for Surface Matching in Neuronavigation. *Comput. Aided Surg.* **2011**, *16*, 161–169. [CrossRef]
28. Hartkens, T.; Hill, D.L.G.; Castellano-Smith, A.D.; Hawkes, D.J.; Maurer, C.R.; Martin, A.J.; Hall, W.A.; Liu, H.; Truwit, C.L. Measurement and Analysis of Brain Deformation during Neurosurgery. *IEEE Trans. Med. Imaging* **2003**, *22*, 82–92. [CrossRef] [PubMed]
29. Stummer, W.; Tonn, J.-C.; Goetz, C.; Ullrich, W.; Stepp, H.; Bink, A.; Pietsch, T.; Pichlmeier, U. 5-Aminolevulinic Acid-Derived Tumor Fluorescence: The Diagnostic Accuracy of Visible Fluorescence Qualities as Corroborated by Spectrometry and Histology and Postoperative Imaging. *Neurosurgery* **2014**, *74*, 310. [CrossRef] [PubMed]
30. Roder, C.; Stummer, W.; Coburger, J.; Scherer, M.; Haas, P.; von der Brelie, C.; Kamp, M.A.; Löhr, M.; Hamisch, C.A.; Skardelly, M.; et al. Intraoperative MRI-Guided Resection Is Not Superior to 5-Aminolevulinic Acid Guidance in Newly Diagnosed Glioblastoma: A Prospective Controlled Multicenter Clinical Trial. *J. Clin. Oncol.* **2023**, *41*, 5512–5523. [CrossRef]
31. Zhang, G.; Li, Z.; Si, D.; Shen, L. Diagnostic Ability of Intraoperative Ultrasound for Identifying Tumor Residual in Glioma Surgery Operation. *Oncotarget* **2017**, *8*, 73105–73114. [CrossRef] [PubMed]
32. Wu, H.; Cheng, Y.; Gao, W.; Chen, P.; Wei, Y.; Zhao, H.; Wang, F. Progress in the Application of Ultrasound in Glioma Surgery. *Front. Med.* **2024**, *11*, 1388728. [CrossRef] [PubMed]
33. Della Pepa, G.M.; Ius, T.; La Rocca, G.; Gaudino, S.; Isola, M.; Pignotti, F.; Rapisarda, A.; Mazzucchi, E.; Giordano, C.; Dragonetti, V.; et al. 5-Aminolevulinic Acid and Contrast-Enhanced Ultrasound: The Combination of the Two Techniques to Optimize the Extent of Resection in Glioblastoma Surgery. *Neurosurgery* **2020**, *86*, E529–E540. [CrossRef]

34. Barbagallo, G.; Maione, M.; Peschillo, S.; Signorelli, F.; Visocchi, M.; Sortino, G.; Fiumanò, G.; Certo, F. Intraoperative Computed Tomography, Navigated Ultrasound, 5-Amino-Levulinic Acid Fluorescence and Neuromonitoring in Brain Tumor Surgery: Overtreatment or Useful Tool Combination? *J. Neurosurg. Sci.* **2019**, *68*, 31–43. [CrossRef] [PubMed]
35. Grasso, E.; Certo, F.; Bonomo, G.; Rossitto, M.; Cammarata, G.; Vitaliti, C.; Barbagallo, G. Role of Virtual iMRI in Glioblastoma Surgery: Advantages, Limitations and Correlation with iCT and Brainshift. *Brain Spine* **2024**, *4*, 103851. [CrossRef]

brain sciences

Article

The Impact of Intraoperative CT-Based Navigation in Congenital Craniovertebral Junction Anomalies: New Concepts of Treatment

Giorgio Cracchiolo [1,2], Ali Baram [3], Gabriele Capo [3], Zefferino Rossini [3], Marco Riva [3,4], Andrea Fanti [2], Mario De Robertis [3], Maurizio Fornari [3], Federico Pessina [3,4] and Carlo Brembilla [3,*]

1 School of Medicine and Surgery, University of Milano-Bicocca, 24127 Bergamo, Bergamo, Italy; g.cracchiolo@campus.unimib.it
2 Department of Neurosurgery, ASST Papa Giovanni XXIII, 24127 Bergamo, Bergamo, Italy; fanti.andrea@gmail.com
3 Department of Neurosurgery, IRCSS Humanitas Research Hospital, Via Alessandro Manzoni 56, 20089 Rozzano, Milan, Italy; ali.baram@humanitas.it (A.B.); gabriele.capo@humanitas.it (G.C.); zefferino.rossini@humanitas.it (Z.R.); marco.riva@hunimed.eu (M.R.); mario.derobertis@humanitas.it (M.D.R.); maurizio.fornari@humanitas.it (M.F.); federico.pessina@hunimed.eu (F.P.)
4 Department of Biomedical Sciences, Humanitas University, Via Rita Levi Montalcini 4, 20090 Pieve Emanuele, Milan, Italy
* Correspondence: carlo.brembilla@humanitas.it or carlinobrembo@gmail.com

Abstract: Background: Congenital craniovertebral junction anomalies (CCVJAs) encompass a diverse range of conditions characterized by distorted anatomy and significant variation in the pathways of neurovascular structures. This study aims to assess the safety and feasibility of tailoring posterior fixation for CCVJAs through intraoperative CT-based navigation. Methods: An in-depth retrospective analysis was conducted on eight patients diagnosed with CCVJAs (excluding Arnold–Chiari malformation). These patients underwent posterior fixation/arthrodesis facilitated by intraoperative CT-based navigation. The analysis included an examination of the fixation strategies, complication rates, length of stay, post-operative complications, and success of arthrodesis. Additionally, a comprehensive literature review was undertaken to contextualize and compare our findings. Results: Patients undergoing CVJ posterior fixation with intraoperative CT-based navigation exhibited a flawless record, devoid of complications related to the damage to neurovascular structures, as well as any instances of screw misposition, pullout, or breakage (0 out of 36 total screws). Furthermore, the entire cohort demonstrated a 100% arthrodesis rate. None of the patients required treatment with an occipital plate. Conclusions: The incorporation of intraoperative CT-based navigation proves to be an invaluable asset in executing CVJ posterior fixation within the context of CCVJAs. This technology facilitates the customization of posterior constructs, a crucial adaptation required to navigate the anatomical challenges posed by these anomalies. The secure placement of screws into the occipital condyles, made possible by navigation, has proven highly effective in achieving CVJ fixation, obviating the need for an occipital plate. This technological leap represents a significant advancement, enhancing the safety, precision, and overall outcomes for patients undergoing this surgical procedure, while concurrently reducing the necessity for more invasive and morbid interventions.

Keywords: craniovertebral junction anomalies; navigation; intraoperative imaging; surgical safety; surgical accuracy; posterior fixation

1. Introduction

The craniovertebral junction (CVJ) serves as a critical anatomical nexus connecting the skull and the cervical spine. This biomechanically complex area includes the occipital condyles (C0), the atlas (C1), the axis (C2), and a network of ligaments crucial for stability, making it the most dynamic part of the cervical spine [1,2].

Since the landmark publication by Goel and Laheri in 1994, which introduced contemporary surgical approaches to this region, the management of CVJ pathologies has evolved significantly [3]. Congenital craniovertebral junction anomalies (CCVJAs) encompass a diverse spectrum of diseases, often characterized by the coexistence of multiple pathologies, presenting significant challenges due to their intricate anatomy [4,5]. These anomalies alter normal anatomical landmarks, potentially leading to confusion during surgery and making the fixation of the region complex and risky for patients [6].

In recent years, technological advancements have transformed the landscape of CCVJA treatment. One particularly important development has been the integration of neuronavigation systems with intraoperative CT scanning. The combination of these technologies has significantly improved the precision and reliability of surgical navigation, allowing for the creation of customized fixation constructs tailored to each patient's unique anatomy. This approach enhances safety while minimizing the need for more invasive procedures [7,8].

To evaluate the safety and feasibility of using intraoperative CT-based navigation for posterior fixation in CCVJAs, we conducted a retrospective analysis of consecutive patients over a 5-year period at a single institution. In addition, we performed a literature review to compare and contextualize our findings.

2. Materials and Methods

2.1. Patient Information

For this study, we selected a cohort of 8 complex congenital craniovertebral junction anomaly (CCVJA) cases treated between 2018 and 2023. The cohort included 7 male patients and 1 female patient, with a mean age of 54 years (range: 4 to 78 years). Diagnoses for the 8 cases are detailed in Table 1, based on Menezes classification [9]. The anomalies in this cohort primarily impacted bone tissue. Surgical intervention was performed due to spinal cord or brainstem compression, CVJ instability, and symptoms such as neck pain, as well as neurological deficits including motor weakness, sensory disturbances, and gait or coordination abnormalities.

Table 1. Summary of 8 patients with craniovertebral junction anomalies.

No.	Age(y)/Sex	Main Radiologic Findings	Instrumentation Choice	Complications	Follow-Up (mo)	Fusion Grade
1	59/F	AA, BI	C0/C1–C2 (Laminar) + Bilateral cages	NA	58	1
2	4/M	DA, BA, BI	C1–C2–C3 (articular)	NA	46	1
3	49/M	OO, AAD	C1–C2	NA	35	1
4	61/M	AA, BI, PB	C0/C1–C2	NA	30	1
5	76/M	OO	C1–C2 fixation + subaxial laminoplasty	NA	24	1
6	78/M	AA, AAD	C0/C1–C2–C3 (pedicular)	Dorsal cervicotoracic hematoma	20	1
7	54/M	OO, AAD	C1–C2 + Jazz™ Lock system	NA	16	1
8	54/M	BA, KF, Odontoid Fracture (Type 3 Anderson-D'Alonzo)	C1–C3 (pedicular)	NA	12	1

AA indicates atlas assimilation; BI, basilar invagination; PB, platybasia; OO, os odontoideum; AAD, atlantoaxial dislocation; BA, bifid ventral and dorsal C1 arches; KF, Klippel–Feil syndrome; DA, dens agenesis; NA, not applicable; C0/C1, occipital condyle/lateral mass fixation; C2, axis; C3, third cervical vertebra.

Arnold–Chiari syndrome was excluded from this series because it is classified as a soft tissue anomaly and often does not necessitate stabilization treatment [10].

2.2. Pre-Operative Planning

CT scans and MRI were pivotal in understanding the nature of CCVJAs by delineating anomalous anatomy, identifying potential dislocation of bony structures, and assessing static spinal cord compression. CT scans allowed for the evaluation of anatomical and physical constraints that could impede conventional screw placement, enabling strategic planning for alternative fixation techniques such as C2 laminar screws. Additionally, CT scans provided valuable information about bone quality [11].

Occipital plates were not considered during the planning phase. In cases where occipitocervical stabilization was required, the strategy involved placing screws in C0 or the hybrid C0/C1 condyle, particularly in cases of atlas assimilation.

Dynamic imaging techniques, including MRI and X-ray, played a crucial role in instability assessment, deformity reducibility, and dynamic compression during neck flexion and extension [12]. CT angiography (CTA) or MR angiography (MRA) were essential for mapping the course of the vertebral arteries (VAs), particularly in patients with CCVJAs, where an aberrant VA course is common [6].

2.3. Surgical Procedure

Patients were placed in the prone position, and their heads were securely placed in the Mayfield head clamp following gentle traction and reduction maneuvers. The intraoperative CT scan (Medtronic O-arm™ Navigation System, Littleton, MA, USA) and the reference frame for navigation were then prepared.

The incision and exposure of the bony elements were performed according to the standard procedure. Huang et al. [13] highlighted the increased risk of post-operative numbness associated with sacrificing the C2 nerve root, while preserving it may lead to neuralgia. In our practice, ligation and sacrifice of the C2 nerve roots represent the standard of care.

The entry point for the C1 lateral mass screw was determined based on the preservation of normal anatomical landmarks and the extent of anatomical distortion. Bicortical screws were preferred to ensure strong anchorage, while the screw length was carefully chosen to avoid inadvertent damage to the internal carotid artery [14]. In cases of atlas assimilation, where the fused C0–C1 vertebrae exhibited hybrid characteristics, the screw trajectory was carefully monitored to ensure clearance of the aberrant course of the VA and/or the hypoglossal nerve. A typical C1 lateral mass screw had a diameter of 3.5 to 4.0 mm and a length of approximately 36 mm [15].

C2 screws offered versatile placement options, including the pars, pedicles, or laminae [16]. In cases with minimal anatomical distortion, C2 pedicle screws were preferred, typically with a diameter of 3.5 mm and lengths ranging from 15 mm to 30 mm [16]. However, when conditions were unfavorable for C2 pedicle screw fixation, alternative techniques were used, with screws positioned in the pars or laminae. For translaminar screw fixation, a crossed trajectory through the laminae of C2 was employed [17,18]. When C2 fixation was not possible or additional stability was required, C3 pedicle or lateral mass screw fixation was performed.

Arthrodesis presented a significant challenge, due to the limited available bone surfaces. Potential bone graft harvesting sites included the posterior iliac crests and the external diploe of the calvarium [19]. To secure the bone graft onto the posterior elements, classic wiring techniques such as Gallie or Brooks–Jenkins were used, which could also be applied to the occiput by drilling holes into the occipital squama [20–22]. Modern solutions like the Jazz™ Lock system, using sublaminar bands, were also utilized. Another technique involved intra-articular arthrodesis between the facet joints of C1 or C0/C1 and C2, which required decorticating the facet joints and filling them with autologous bone chips and/or synthetic bone substitute. In cases where intra-articular gap widening occurred during reduction, the atlantoaxial joint jamming technique was applied, involving the placement of bilateral interbody fusion cages and bone graft material in the intra-articular spaces to ensure biomechanical stability for fusion [23,24].

2.4. Complication Avoidance and Follow-Up

Thorough evaluation of pre-operative imaging was crucial for assessing the precise location and abnormal paths of the VAs. The VA is particularly vulnerable to injury during soft tissue dissection around the C1 posterior arch, the placement of C0/C1 screws in cases of atlas assimilation, and the insertion of C2 pedicle screws. Although the hypoglossal canal is typically described as a supracondylar structure, its trajectory may be altered in the context of CCVJAs, increasing the risk of injury during screw insertion [6,25,26].

In cases where pre-operative evaluation revealed significant spinal cord compression or compromise of neural structures, the surgical procedure was performed with intraoperative neurophysiological monitoring, as seen in patients 2 and 7.

Following surgery, patients were immobilized with a rigid cervical collar starting from the first post-operative day for approximately one month, followed by a rehabilitation phase during the subsequent month. Clinical follow-up monitored medium- and long-term complications. Imaging follow-up involved cervical spine CT scans at 1, 3, 6, and 12 months, and then annually. Fusion was evaluated based on the criteria outlined by Tan et al. [27], focusing on documenting bridging osseous union between the proximal and distal endpoints. All patients underwent both imaging and clinical follow-up for a minimum of 12 months.

2.5. Search Strategy and Eligibility

A systematic search was conducted across SCOPUS, Medline (PubMed), Cochrane Library, and Google Scholar databases to identify all studies providing relevant information on the use of intraoperative CT scans coupled with navigation in the posterior treatment of CCVJAs. There were no date limits or language restrictions applied during the search. Various combinations of key terms such as "craniovertebral junction anomalies", "posterior fixation", and "intraoperative neuronavigation" were used. Additionally, a thorough examination of the references in all included articles was conducted to identify any additional eligible studies. The review included all peer-reviewed case series that reported on the use of intraoperative navigation for the posterior fixation of CCVJAs. Exclusion criteria were as follows: (1) letters to editors and conference abstracts, (2) studies reporting on the use of intraoperative navigation for anterior approaches to the CVJ, (3) studies on the use of intraoperative navigation for posterior fixation of non-malformed vertebrae, and (4) studies on posterior fixation of CCVJAs without the use of intraoperative neuronavigation.

3. Results

3.1. Surgical Case Series

Intraoperative CT scans with neuronavigation were successfully used for the posterior fixation of eight cases of CCVJAs. All patients underwent rod and screw fixation, with specific techniques tailored to each case. C0/C1 fixation was performed in three cases, C1 lateral mass fixation in five cases, C2 pedicle screw fixation in six cases, and C2 translaminar screw fixation in one case (patient 1). Additionally, C3 pedicle screw fixation was performed in two cases (patients 6 and 8), C3 lateral mass fixation in one case (patient 2), and bilateral 5 mm interbody cages were placed in the C1–C2 articular spaces in one case (patient 1). The Jazz™ Lock system was used in one case (patient 7). Autografts were used in two cases (patients 4 and 7). In all eight cases, correct screw placement and malformation reduction were achieved without injury to the vascular or neural structures. There were no intraoperative or post-operative screw replacements (0 out of 36 screws) due to mispositioning, pullout, or breakage. The average intraoperative surgical time was 209 min. In the immediate post-operative period, one case (patient 6) experienced a dorsal cervicothoracic hematoma on the 14th post-operative day. The average length of stay following surgery was 12 days. The average intraoperative time and length of stay were influenced by patient 8, a polytraumatized patient who underwent multiple surgical interventions in the same session. During the follow-up period, one patient (patient 1) experienced a mild reduction loss without clinical consequences. Arthrodesis was achieved in seven out of eight cases, and osteosynthesis in one case (patient 8), with all eight cases classified as grade I fusions according to Tan et al. [27].

3.2. Study Identification

After conducting an extensive database search, we identified two relevant studies. Despite a thorough examination of references, no additional studies were found. One study was excluded from the review as it did not meet the eligibility criteria; it focused on assessing the utility of intraoperative neuronavigation for a bony resection through anterior approaches to the malformed CVJ [28]. The included study, published in 2014, was a Chinese case series involving 23 patients with CCVJAs, all treated with posterior fixation using intraoperative CT and neuronavigation [29]. The authors reported an overall accuracy rate of 98.1%, with only two misplaced screws, and a 100% arthrodesis rate, without any neurovascular complications. Notably, ten patients underwent occipitocervical fixation using an occipital plate, either due to C1 hypoplasia or limitations imposed by the C2 bone structure.

3.3. Illustrative Cases

Case 1 (Figure 1)

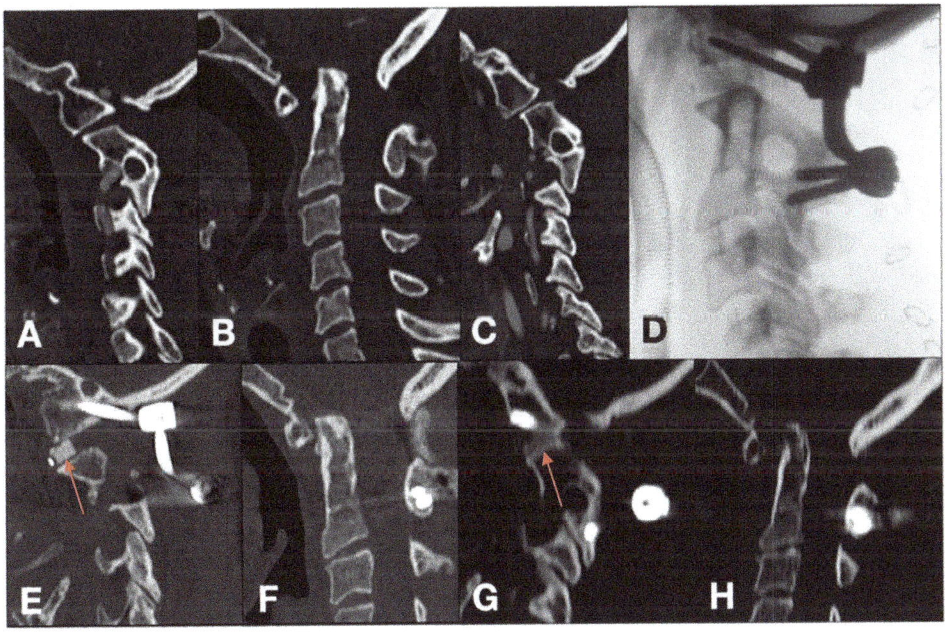

Figure 1. Pre-operative sagittal CT scan (**A–C**). Intra-operative radiographic acquisition (**D**). Three-month follow-up CT scan demonstrating correct intra-articular cage positioning (red arrow) and reduction in the malformation (**E**,**F**). 58-month follow-up CT scans demonstrating C0/C1-C2 arthrodesis achievement (red arrow) and mild loss of reduction (**G**,**H**).

A 59-year-old female with a history of chronic hemicrania and severe neck pain was presented at our institution. A CT scan revealed basilar invagination with a dysmorphic dens, along with atlas assimilation. A dynamic MRI confirmed the diagnosis of basilar invagination and assessed the reducibility of the malformation. During positioning, after a distraction and reduction in the malformation, an intraoperative radiograph showed a 6 mm separation between the C0/C1 and C2 facet joints. Our intervention involved decorticating the C0/C1 and C2 facet joints, followed by placing two bilateral 6 mm cages filled with calcium triphosphate (PEEK interbody device; Cervios, DepuySynthes, Raynham, MA, USA). C0/C1 lateral mass-condyle fixation (3.5 $\times$ 30 mm) and C2 translaminar fixation (3.5 $\times$ 30 mm) were used as anchorage points. After placing the rods, a synthetic bone allograft was applied over the construct. A follow-up CT scan at 58 months showed a mild loss of correction but confirmed the successful arthrodesis at the affected segment.

Case 2 (Figure 2)

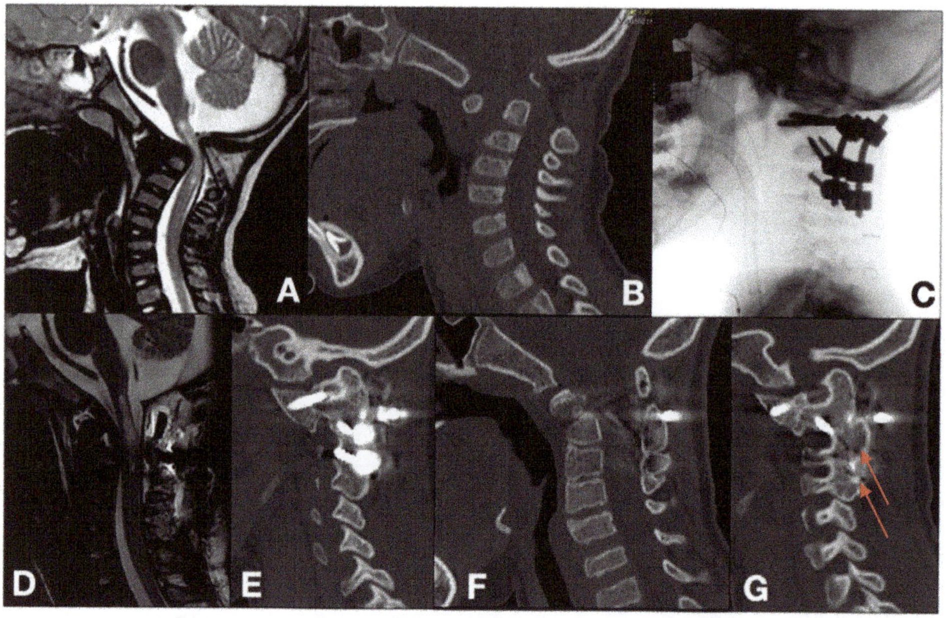

Figure 2. Pre-operative T2-weighted sagittal MRI scan (**A**). Pre-operative sagittal CT scan (**B**). Intra-operative radiographic acquisition (**C**). Post-operative T2-weighted sagittal MRI scan (**D**). 46-month follow-up sagittal CT scan demonstrating correct alignment, reduction in the malformation, and arthrodesis achievement (red arrows) (**E**–**G**).

A 4-year-old male was presented to our emergency department with progressive tetraparesis. An MRI scan revealed CCVJAs, characterized by basilar invagination along with dens agenesis. T2-weighted sequences showed the spinal cord hyperintensity and a syringomyelic cavity extending from the brainstem to C2. Subsequent CT scans confirmed the MRI findings, highlighting the bifid ventral and dorsal arches of C1, dens agenesis leading to C1–C2 instability, and severe segmental kyphosis. A partial reduction in the dislocation was achieved under fluoroscopic guidance by applying a halo vest, which was maintained for 15 consecutive days with progressively increased traction to enhance reduction. Posterior fixation and arthrodesis were performed with intraoperative neuromonitoring. C1 lateral mass fixation (28 mm length), C2 pedicle fixation (16 mm length), and C3 lateral mass fixation (8 mm length) were established as anchorage points. Rigorous reduction maneuvers, facilitated by rod positioning and securing, resulted in good cervical alignment. A synthetic bone allograft was applied over the surgical site to close the C1 dorsal cleft and promote C1–C3 arthrodesis. A follow-up CT scan at 46 months demonstrated the successful arthrodesis of the C1–C2–C3 segment, closure of the C1 dorsal cleft, and maintenance of the reduction achieved intraoperatively. The patient is now able to walk independently, with a slight tendency toward the internal rotation of the feet and mild motor weakness in the upper limbs.

Case 4 (Figure 3)

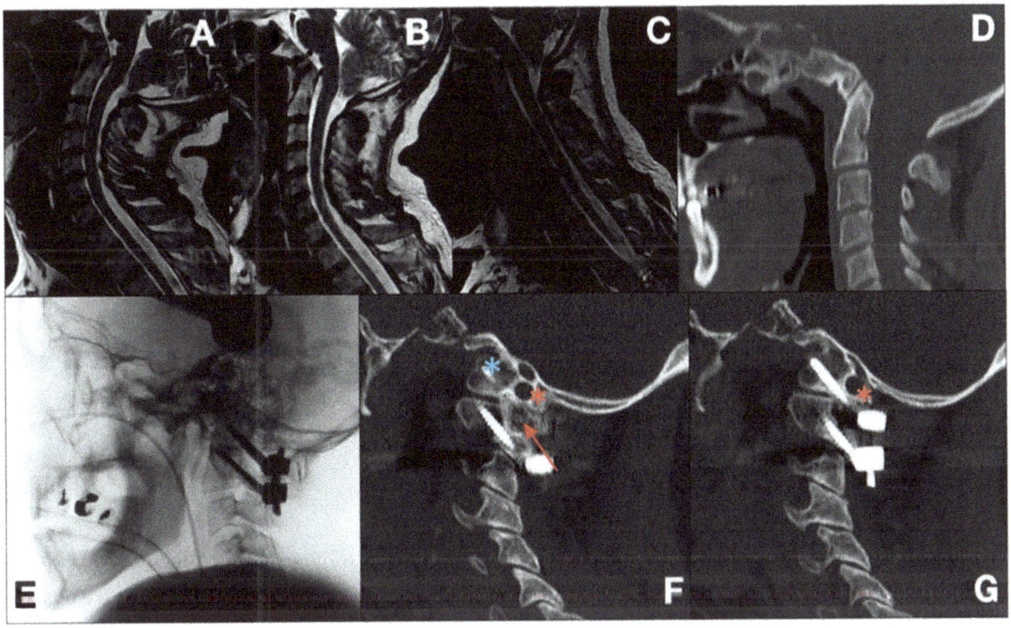

Figure 3. Pre-operative T2-weighted extension, neutral, and flexion sagittal MRI scans, respectively (**A–C**). Pre-operative sagittal CT scan (**D**). Intra-operative radiographic acquisition (**E**). 30-month follow-up sagittal CT scans demonstrating correct alignment, arthrodesis achievement (red arrow), and correct screw insertion avoiding critical neurovascular structures (red asterisk for vascular structures and blue asterisk for neural structures) (**F,G**).

A 61-year-old male was presented to our institution with severe and progressively worsening neck pain, along with left-sided brachiocrural hemiparesis that varied with head position. These symptoms developed following two previous head traumas. A CT scan revealed atlas assimilation, basilar invagination, and platybasia. A subsequent dynamic MRI confirmed the basilar invagination, showing a dynamic conflict between the basilar artery/brainstem and the tip of the C2 dens, as well as instability of the left C1–C2 joint. To address these issues, posterior fixation and arthrodesis were performed, using C0/C1 lateral mass-condyle screws (3.5 × 26 mm) and C2 pedicle screws (3.5 × 30 mm) as anchorage points. After placing and securing the rods, an autologous bone graft was harvested from the external diploe of the calvarium. This graft was then secured to the instrumentation using non-resorbable braided sutures, creating an arthrodesis bed between the assimilated C1 arch and the C2 lamina. The patient experienced a complete resolution of symptoms, and a follow-up CT scan at 30 months confirmed the successful CVJ arthrodesis.

Case 8 (Figure 4)

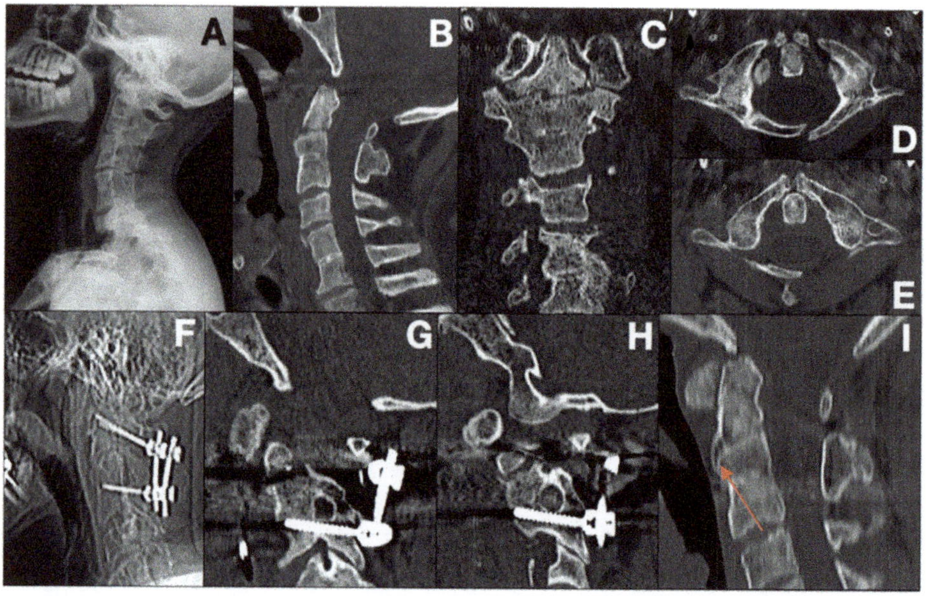

Figure 4. Pre-operative radiographic acquisition (**A**). Pre-operative sagittal, coronal, and axial CT scans, respectively (**B–E**). Intra-operative radiographic acquisition (**F**). 12-month follow-up sagittal CT scans demonstrating osteosynthesis achievement (red arrow) and correct screw alignment in the C3 peduncles (**G–I**).

A 45-year-old male with a history of substance abuse (alcohol, cocaine, and psychiatric drugs) and HCV positivity was brought to our emergency department after being struck by a bus. The patient displayed no neurological deficits. A cervical spine CT revealed multiple conditions, including bifid ventral and dorsal arches of C1, Klippel–Feil syndrome at C2–C3 and C5–C6, a Type 3 Anderson–D'Alonzo odontoid fracture at C2, and a left lateral mass fracture at C2. Due to the limited size of the C2 pedicles, C1 lateral mass fixation (3.5 × 34 mm screws) and C3 pedicle fixation (3.5 × 26 mm screws) were selected as anchorage points. A follow-up CT scan at 12 months demonstrated ongoing osteosynthesis, evidenced by the formation of bony trabeculae along the previously fractured lines.

4. Discussion

4.1. Background

The CVJ is a complex structure involving bones, joints, ligaments, and neurovascular components [30]. Congenital anomalies can alter the biomechanics of this region, leading to instability and biomechanical overload [31,32]. Posterior atlantoaxial fixation (AA) is essential for managing CVJ conditions, and techniques have evolved over time, although concerns such as VA injury remain [33,34]. Goel and Harms [5,35–38] introduced techniques that allow individual screw placement, reducing anatomical limitations and the risk of VA injury. Various options, including C2 pedicle, pars, and translaminar screws, have been developed to balance screw anchoring with VA safety [17,39].

In cases of hypoplastic C1 or C1 assimilation, surgeons have historically opted for occipitocervical fixation, often using an occipital plate. However, this approach is associated with complications, such as hardware prominence and a high rate of pseudoarthrosis [40], prompting the exploration of alternatives like occipital condyle (C0) fixation [25,41]. Although these approaches offer increased stiffness and a reduced range of motion, they still carry risks, particularly in patients with CCVJAs.

4.2. Advancements

The introduction of intraoperative navigation has significantly improved screw insertion success rates while reducing complications. Intraoperative neuronavigation provides a three-dimensional virtual map that merges imaging data with real-time intraoperative visualization. This enhances the surgeon's ability to plan accurate trajectories, minimize the risk of iatrogenic injury, and improve overall surgical precision [42–44].

The surgical series presented here highlights the practical applications and advantages of intraoperative navigation in posterior fixation for CCVJAs. The technology played a crucial role in guiding surgical decisions, enabling precise trajectory planning, and contributing to successful outcomes. It was particularly effective in preventing damage to the VA and hypoglossal nerve during fixation, even in cases where it was preferred over occipital fixation.

The benefits also extended to C2 and C3 pedicle screw fixation, reducing surgical time, blood loss, and complication rates. The outcomes of this study align with those reported by Yu et al., further reinforcing the reliability of intraoperative navigation [29].

4.3. Limitations

Despite the advantages, certain limitations must be acknowledged. These include the potential for registration errors, image distortion, and system malfunctions. [45–47]. Surgeons must maintain proficiency in interpreting and integrating navigation system data while exercising sound clinical judgment. Accessibility and cost may also present challenges in resource-limited settings, requiring the careful evaluation of feasibility and cost-effectiveness.

The specific limitations of this study include a small patient cohort, the absence of a control group, and a relatively short follow-up duration for some individuals. However, the variability within the pathologies demonstrated the value of navigation in adapting to diverse cases, enabling customized constructs tailored to specific anatomical intricacies.

5. Conclusions

In conclusion, our case series and comprehensive literature review highlight the transformative impact of intraoperative navigation on posterior fixation in CCVJAs, representing a significant advancement in surgical precision. Despite challenges related to technical aspects and cost considerations, the advantages of intraoperative navigation are setting a new standard in CCVJA treatment. This technology enables the customization of posterior constructs, a crucial adaptation for addressing anatomical challenges and reducing perioperative neurovascular complications.

In our case series, the effective use of navigation for secure screw placement in the occipital condyles has proven successful in treating CCVJAs, eliminating the need for an occipital plate. Traditionally, occipitocervical constructs that include an occipital plate have been associated with lower fusion rates and increased complication risks. These improvements represent a substantial leap forward, enhancing the safety, precision, and overall outcomes of surgeries in this field, while reducing the need for more invasive and burdensome interventions. As intraoperative navigation becomes increasingly integral, it heralds a new era in the treatment of CCVJAs, offering tailored solutions that address the unique challenges posed by these anomalies.

Author Contributions: C.B. and G.C. (Giorgio Cracchiolo) conceived of the presented idea, and wrote the main manuscript text. A.F., G.C. (Giorgio Cracchiolo), A.B., M.D.R., M.R., M.F., F.P., Z.R. and G.C. (Gabriele Capo). collected the data, and prepared the figures and Table 1. All authors discussed the design and contributed to the final manuscript. C.B. and G.C. (Giorgio Cracchiolo) supervised the project. All authors have read and agreed to the published version of the manuscript.

Funding: This research received no external funding.

Institutional Review Board Statement: The ethical review and approval were waived for this study because it involves procedures considered standard clinical practice and routinely performed at our institution. These procedures, including personalized screw positioning and vertebral level selection using intraoperative CT-based navigation, are part of the established treatment protocols for patients with congenital craniovertebral junction anomalies. The decision to use these techniques was made solely based on clinical judgement and patient needs, independent of study inclusion. No modifications to standard care were made for research purposes.

Informed Consent Statement: Informed consent was obtained from all subjects involved in the study.

Data Availability Statement: We excluded the data availability section since our study did not report on any data present in public datasets.

Conflicts of Interest: The authors declare no conflicts of interest.

Abbreviations

The following abbreviations are used in this manuscript:

CCVJA	congenital craniovertebral junction anomalies
CVJ	craniovertebral junction
VA	vertebral artery

References

1. White, A.A., 3rd; Panjabi, M.M. The clinical biomechanics of the occipitoatlantoaxial complex. *Orthop. Clin. N. Am.* **1978**, *9*, 867–878. [CrossRef]
2. Menezes, A.H.; Traynelis, V.C. Anatomy and biomechanics of normal craniovertebral junction (a) and biomechanics of stabilization (b). *Childs Nerv. Syst.* **2008**, *24*, 1091–1100. [CrossRef] [PubMed]
3. Goel, A.; Laheri, V. Plate and screw fixation for atlanto-axial subluxation. *Acta Neurochir* **1994**, *129*, 47–53. [CrossRef] [PubMed]
4. Erbengi, A.; Oge, H.K. Congenital malformations of the craniovertebral junction: Classification and surgical treatment. *Acta Neurochir.* **1994**, *127*, 180–185. [CrossRef]
5. Du, J.; Gao, X.; Huang, Y.; Yang, X.; Zheng, B.; Liu, Z.; Hui, H.; Gao, L.; Wu, J.; Zhao, Z.; et al. Posterior Surgery in the Treatment of Craniovertebral Junction Deformity with Torticollis. *Orthop. Surg.* **2022**, *14*, 2418–2426. [CrossRef]
6. Yamazaki, M.; Koda, M.; Aramomi, M.A.; Hashimoto, M.; Masaki, Y.; Okawa, A. Anomalous vertebral artery at the extraosseous and intraosseous regions of the craniovertebral junction: Analysis by three-dimensional computed tomography angiography. *Spine* **2005**, *30*, 2452–2457. [CrossRef]
7. Holly, L.T.; Foley, K.T. Intraoperative spinal navigation. *Spine* **2003**, *28* (Suppl. S15), S54–S61. [CrossRef]
8. Oertel, M.F.; Hobart, J.; Stein, M.; Schreiber, V.; Scharbrodt, W. Clinical and methodological precision of spinal navigation assisted by 3D intraoperative O-arm radiographic imaging. *J. Neurosurg. Spine* **2011**, *14*, 532–536. [CrossRef]
9. Menezes, A.H. Congenital and acquired abnormalities of the craniovertebral junction (children and adults). In *Neurological Surgery*; Youmans, J., Ed.; WB Saunders: Philadelphia, PA, USA, 1995; pp. 1035–1089.
10. Ravikanth, R.; Majumdar, P. Embryological considerations and evaluation of congenital anomalies of craniovertebral junction: A single-center experience. *Tzu Chi Med. J.* **2020**, *33*, 175–180. [CrossRef]
11. Wang, M.Y.; Samudrala, S. Cadaveric morphometric analysis for atlantal lateral mass screw placement. *Neurosurgery* **2004**, *54*, 1436–1439, discussion 1439–1440. [CrossRef]
12. Michelini, G.; Corridore, A.; Torlone, S.; Bruno, F.; Marsecano, C.; Capasso, R.; Caranci, F.; Barile, A.; Masciocchi, C.; Splendiani, A. Dynamic MRI in the evaluation of the spine: State of the art. *Acta Biomed.* **2018**, *89*, 89–101. [PubMed]
13. Huang, D.G.; Hao, D.J.; Li, G.L.; Guo, H.; Zhang, Y.C.; He, B.R. C2 nerve dysfunction associated with C1 lateral mass screw fixation. *Orthop. Surg.* **2014**, *6*, 269–273. [CrossRef] [PubMed]
14. Currier, B.L.; Todd, L.T.; Maus, T.P.; Fisher, D.R.; Yaszemski, M.J. Anatomic relationship of the internal carotid artery to the C1 vertebra: A case report of cervical reconstruction for chordoma and pilot study to assess the risk of screw fixation of the atlas. *Spine* **2003**, *28*, E461–E467. [CrossRef] [PubMed]
15. Fiore, A.J.; Haid, R.W.; Rodts, G.E.; Subach, B.R.; Mummaneni, P.V.; Riedel, C.J.; Birch, B.D. Atlantal lateral mass screws for posterior spinal reconstruction: Technical note and case series. *Neurosurg. Focus* **2002**, *12*, E5. [CrossRef] [PubMed]
16. Bydon, A.; Xu, R.; Bydon, M.; Macki, M.; Belkoff, S.; Langdale, E.; McGovern, K.; Wolinsky, J.-P.; Gokalsan, Z. Biomechanical impact of C2 pedicle screw length in an atlantoaxial fusion construct. *Surg. Neurol. Int.* **2014**, *5* (Suppl. S7), S343–S346. [CrossRef]
17. Huang, D.-G.; Hao, D.-J.; He, B.-R.; Wu, Q.-N.; Liu, T.-J.; Wang, X.-D.; Guo, H.; Fang, X.-Y. Posterior atlantoaxial fixation: A review of all techniques. *Spine J.* **2015**, *15*, 2271–2281. [CrossRef]
18. Chin, K.R.; Mills, M.V.; Seale, J.; Cumming, V. Ideal starting point and trajectory for C2 pedicle screw placement: A 3D computed tomography analysis using perioperative measurements. *Spine J.* **2014**, *14*, 615–618. [CrossRef]
19. Jakoi, A.M.; Iorio, J.A.; Cahill, P.J. Autologous bone graft harvesting: A review of grafts and surgical techniques. *Musculoskelet. Surg.* **2015**, *99*, 171–178. [CrossRef]
20. Gallie, W.E. Fractures and dislocations of the cervical spine. *Am. J. Surg.* **1939**, *46*, 495–499. [CrossRef]

21. Brooks, A.L.; Jenkins, E.B. Atlanto-axial arthrodesis by the wedge compression method. *J. Bone Jt. Surg. Am.* **1978**, *60*, 279–284. [CrossRef]
22. Dickman, C.A.; Sonntag, V.K.; Papadopoulos, S.M.; Hadley, M.N. The interspinous method of posterior atlantoaxial arthrodesis. *J. Neurosurg.* **1991**, *74*, 190–198. [CrossRef] [PubMed]
23. Goel, A. Atlantoaxial joint jamming as a treatment for atlantoaxial dislocation: A preliminary report: Technical note. *J. Neurosurg. Spine* **2007**, *7*, 90–94. [CrossRef] [PubMed]
24. Gelinne, A.; Piazza, M.; Bhowmick, D.A. Minimally invasive modification of the Goel-Harms atlantoaxial fusion technique: A case series and illustrative guide. *Neurosurg. Focus* **2023**, *54*, E14. [CrossRef] [PubMed]
25. Uribe, J.S.; Ramos, E.; Youssef, A.S.; Levine, N.; Turner, A.W.; Johnson, W.M.; Vale, F.L. Craniocervical fixation with occipital condyle screws: Biomechanical analysis of a novel technique. *Spine* **2010**, *35*, 931–938. [CrossRef] [PubMed]
26. Jian, F.Z.; Su, C.H.; Chen, Z.; Wang, X.W.; Ling, F. Feasibility and limitations of C1 lateral mass screw placement in patients of atlas assimilation. *Clin. Neurol. Neurosurg.* **2012**, *114*, 590–596. [CrossRef]
27. Tan, G.H.; Goss, B.G.; Thorpe, P.J.; Williams, R.P. CT-based classification of long spinal allograft fusion. *Eur. Spine J.* **2007**, *16*, 1875–1881. [CrossRef]
28. Li, L.; Wang, P.; Chen, L.; Ma, X.; Bu, B.; Yu, X. Individualized treatment of craniovertebral junction malformation guided by intraoperative computed tomography. *J. Spinal Disord. Tech.* **2012**, *25*, 77–84. [CrossRef]
29. Yu, X.; Li, L.; Wang, P.; Yin, Y.; Bu, B.; Zhou, D. Intraoperative computed tomography with an integrated navigation system in stabilization surgery for complex craniovertebral junction malformation. *J. Spinal Disord. Tech.* **2014**, *27*, 245–252. [CrossRef]
30. Lopez, A.J.; Scheer, J.K.; Leibl, K.E.; Smith, Z.A.; Dlouhy, B.J.; Dahdaleh, N.S. Anatomy and biomechanics of the craniovertebral junction. *Neurosurg. Focus* **2015**, *38*, E2. [CrossRef]
31. Samartzis, D.; Shen, F.H.; Herman, J.; Mardjetko, S.M. Atlantoaxial rotatory fixation in the setting of associated congenital malformations: A modified classification system. *Spine* **2010**, *35*, E119–E127. [CrossRef]
32. Panjabi, M.M.; White, A.A., 3rd. Basic biomechanics of the spine. *Neurosurgery* **1980**, *7*, 76–93. [CrossRef] [PubMed]
33. Jeanneret, B.; Magerl, F. Primary posterior fusion C1/2 in odontoid fractures: Indications, technique, and results of transarticular screw fixation. *J. Spinal Disord.* **1992**, *5*, 464–475. [CrossRef] [PubMed]
34. Wright, N.M.; Lauryssen, C. Vertebral artery injury in C1-2 transarticular screw fixation: Results of a survey of the AANS/CNS section on disorders of the spine and peripheral nerves. American Association of Neurological Surgeons/Congress of Neurological Surgeons. *J. Neurosurg.* **1998**, *88*, 634–640. [CrossRef] [PubMed]
35. Goel, A.; Desai, K.I.; Muzumdar, D.P. Atlantoaxial fixation using plate and screw method: A report of 160 treated patients. *Neurosurgery* **2002**, *51*, 1351–1356, discussion 1356–1357. [CrossRef]
36. Goel, A.; Kulkarni, A.G.; Sharma, P. Reduction of fixed atlantoaxial dislocation in 24 cases: Technical note. *J. Neurosurg. Spine* **2005**, *2*, 505–509. [CrossRef]
37. Harms, J.; Melcher, R.P. Posterior C1-C2 fusion with polyaxial screw and rod fixation. *Spine* **2001**, *26*, 2467–2471. [CrossRef]
38. Chun, D.H.; Yoon, D.H.; Kim, K.N.; Yi, S.; Shin, D.A.; Ha, Y. Biomechanical Comparison of Four Different Atlantoaxial Posterior Fixation Constructs in Adults: A Finite Element Study. *Spine* **2018**, *43*, E891–E897. [CrossRef]
39. Chang, C.-C.; Huang, W.-C.; Tu, T.-H.; Chang, P.-Y.; Fay, L.-Y.; Wu, J.-C.; Cheng, H. Differences in fixation strength among constructs of atlantoaxial fixation. *J. Neurosurg. Spine* **2018**, *30*, 52–59. [CrossRef]
40. Joaquim, A.F.; Osorio, J.A.; Riew, K.D. Occipitocervical Fixation: General Considerations and Surgical Technique. *Global Spine J.* **2020**, *10*, 647–656. [CrossRef]
41. Uribe, J.S.; Ramos, E.; Vale, F. Feasibility of occipital condyle screw placement for occipitocervical fixation: A cadaveric study and description of a novel technique. *J. Spinal Disord. Tech.* **2008**, *21*, 540–546. [CrossRef]
42. Rajasekaran, S.; Kanna, P.R.; Shetty, T.A. Intra-operative computer navigation guided cervical pedicle screw insertion in thirty-three complex cervical spine deformities. *J. Craniovertebr. Junction Spine* **2010**, *1*, 38–43. [CrossRef] [PubMed]
43. Kosmopoulos, V.; Schizas, C. Pedicle screw placement accuracy: A meta-analysis. *Spine* **2007**, *32*, E111–E120. [CrossRef] [PubMed]
44. Larson, A.N.; Polly, D.W.J.; Guidera, K.J.; Mielke, C.H.; Santos, E.R.G.; Ledonio, C.G.T.; Sembrano, J.N. The accuracy of navigation and 3D image-guided placement for the placement of pedicle screws in congenital spine deformity. *J. Pediatr. Orthop.* **2012**, *32*, e23–e29. [CrossRef]
45. Mischkowski, R.A.; Zinser, M.J.; Ritter, L.; Neugebauer, J.; Keeve, E.; Zöller, J.E. Intraoperative navigation in the maxillofacial area based on 3D imaging obtained by a cone-beam device. *Int. J. Oral. Maxillofac. Surg.* **2007**, *36*, 687–694. [CrossRef]
46. Dalgorf, D.; Daly, M.; Chan, H.; Siewerdsen, J.; Irish, J. Accuracy and reproducibility of automatic versus manual registration using a cone-beam CT image guidance system. *J. Otolaryngol. Head. Neck Surg.* **2011**, *40*, 75–80.
47. Schicho, K.; Figl, M.; Seemann, R.; Donat, M.; Pretterklieber, M.L.; Birkfellner, W.; Reichwein, A.; Wanschitz, F.; Kainberger, F.; Bergmann, H.; et al. Comparison of laser surface scanning and fiducial marker-based registration in frameless stereotaxy: Technical note. *J. Neurosurg.* **2007**, *106*, 704–709. [CrossRef]

brain sciences

MDPI

Article

Cerebrospinal Fluid Leak Prevention in Intradural Spine Surgery: A Long Series Analysis of Closure with Non-Penetrating Titanium Clips

Leonardo Anselmi [1,2,†], Carla Daniela Anania [1,*,†], Maria Cleofe Ubezio [2], Generoso Farinaro [1,2], Donato Creatura [1,2], Alessandro Ortolina [1], Massimo Tomei [1], Ali Baram [1] and Maurizio Fornari [1]

[1] Department of Neurosurgery, IRCCS Humanitas Research Hospital, Via Manzoni 56, 20089 Rozzano, Italy; leonardo.anselmi@humanitas.it (L.A.); generoso.farinaro@humanitas.it (G.F.); donato.creatura@humanitas.it (D.C.); alessandro.ortolina@humanitas.it (A.O.); massimo.tomei@humanitas.it (M.T.); ali.baram@humanitas.it (A.B.); maurizio.fornari@humanitas.it (M.F.)

[2] Department of Biomedical Sciences, Humanitas University, Via R.L Montalcini 2, 20072 Pieve Emanuele, Italy; mariacleofe.ubezio@st.hunimed.eu

* Correspondence: carla.anania@yahoo.it

† These authors contributed equally to this work.

Abstract: Background/Objectives: Postoperative cerebrospinal fluid (CSF) fistulas remain a significant concern in spinal neurosurgery, particularly following dural closure. The incidence of dural tears during spinal surgery is estimated between 1.6% and 10%. While direct suturing remains the gold standard, it has a failure rate of 5–10%. Various materials and techniques have been used to enhance dural closure. This study aims to assess the effectiveness of non-penetrating titanium clips (AnastoClip®) for dural closure in intradural spinal lesion surgeries. **Methods**: A prospective analysis was conducted on 272 patients who were operated on for intradural spinal lesions from August 2017 to December 2023. Dural closure was performed using non-penetrating titanium clips with sealant, and, in select cases, autologous grafts. Postoperative care included early mobilization and routine MRI to assess outcomes. A comparative analysis was performed with a cohort of 81 patients treated with traditional sutures. **Results**: Among the 272 patients, postoperative CSF leaks occurred in 32 cases (11.76%), requiring various management approaches. Thirteen cases required surgical revision, while others resolved with external lumbar drainage or fluid aspiration. Compared to the suture group, which had a fistula rate of 23.46%, the titanium clip group had a significantly lower fistula rate. Logistic regression analysis did not find statistically significant associations between fistula risk and clinical factors. **Conclusions**: Non-penetrating titanium clips provide an effective alternative to sutures for dural closure, reducing CSF leak rates. They preserve dural integrity, reduce operative time, and avoid imaging artifacts, making them a viable advancement in spinal surgery with outcomes comparable to, or better than, traditional techniques.

Keywords: AnastoClip; non-penetrating titanium clip; durotomy; dural closure; CSF; dural tears; spinal intradural tumors surgery; spine surgery

1. Introduction

Avoiding postoperative cerebrospinal fluid fistulas has been a challenge in neurosurgery for a long time [1]. Dural opening in spinal surgery may be intentional, as in intradural procedures, or incidental, as in dural tears, with dural opening occurring in 1.6% to 10% of cases in other types of spinal surgery [2]. Over time, various methods have been proposed to obtain a watertight closure including different suture techniques (interrupted or continuous) [3] and additional sealing materials and grafts such as autologous fat or muscle [4,5]. Even today, there is no consensus on the most appropriate closure method or postoperative management approach to minimize the risk of dural opening. Nowadays, the primary accepted goal worldwide is to obtain the direct suture whenever possible in order to reduce the cerebrospinal fluid leakage with minimal risk; however, even with additional sealants, the use of direct sutures is still associated with a 5% to 10% failure rate [6].

Over the years, a lot of innovative and alternative methods have been described with the aim of obtaining a watertight closure that could be performed in a safer, easier, and more rapid way. Based on the first studies in 2010 and the more recent paper of Kiyoshi Ito in 2017, we have introduced the use of non-penetrating titanium clips (the AnastoClip® AC Closure System.LeMaitre Vascular S.R.L. Via Clemente Prudenzio 14/16 20138 Milano (MI), Italy) at our department for dural closure in both intentional and incidental durotomy [7]. We collected a series of almost 300 surgical procedures for intradural spinal lesions operated on with this closure technique. We also gathered a prospective collection of all cases to analyze the feasibility and the effectiveness of this novel technique in terms of the prevention of dural fistulas and the reduction of the reintervention rate. To achieve this result, we made a comparison with a retrospective analysis of a series of patients operated on from 2015 to 2017.

In this paper, we present the surgical technique and the results of both the prospective collection and the comparative analysis.

2. Materials and Methods

We prospectively analyzed a series of patients operated on at our Neurosurgery Department from August 2017 to December 2023 for resection of intradural spinal lesions both intra- and extramedullary. The study includes adult patients who underwent resection of intradural spinal tumors with an intact dura mater, where dural closure was achieved using non-penetrating titanium clips. Excluded from the study were patients with a history of prior surgery for intradural spinal lesions, those who experienced incidental durotomy requiring suturing, and patients whose postoperative dural defects necessitated the use of artificial dural patches. All patients underwent the same closure technique and postoperative cares protocol. In detail, dural closure was achieved by the placement of non-penetrating titanium clips (AnastoClip®) and sealant; patches (gelatin sponge or Tachoseal®) or autologous graft (adipose or muscular tissue) were applied in selected cases. Patients deemed at risk were kept in bed for 24 to 48 h, while the majority were mobilized the day after surgery. The surgical technique and postoperative cares protocol are shown in Figure 1 and detailed in Appendix A.

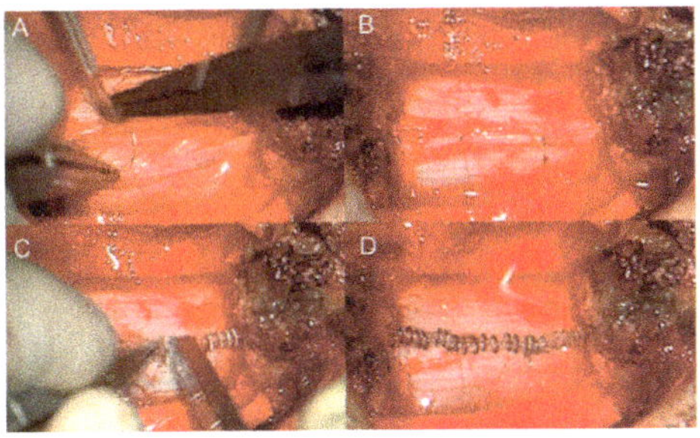

Figure 1. Closure technique for intentional durotomy. For the closure of the dura mater, we use two to three stitches with Prolene 6-0 suture thread and a curved needle: two stitches are placed at the edges of the dural opening, with one or two additional stitches in the middle, depending on the size of the opening (**A**,**B**). Titanium clips are then applied to secure the dural closure, followed by the application of a sealant (**C**,**D**).

Clinical data such as age, sex, BMI, operative data including the size of dural opening (dimensionally equivalent to the number of vertebrae), vertebral segment (divided in cervical, dorsal, lumbar, and sacral), and pathological data such as the histological type of tumor were analyzed. Additionally, the number of fistulas and the method of resolution were evaluated, including reintervention, placement of an external lumbar drainage (ELD) catheter, reintervention plus ELD, or spontaneous resolution after aspiration of the collection and compressive medication. For a comparative analysis, a similar population of patients undergoing dural closure with standard sutures operated on from January 2015 to December 2017, prior to the introduction of clips, was retrospectively analyzed.

To reduce biases, we did not analyze patients with incidental durotomy repaired with titanium clips.

The study was approved by our institutional ethics committee (N° 31/24).

3. Results

We conducted a comprehensive analysis involving 272 patients, encompassing 120 males and 152 females, with a mean age of 56 years (range: 11–89). Within this cohort, 234 individuals presented with extramedullary lesions, 33 with intramedullary lesions, and 5 with combined intra- and extramedullary involvement. Anatomical distribution revealed 57 cervical, 105 thoracic, 108 lumbar, and 2 sacral lesions. Dural exposure ranged from one level in 69 cases, two levels in 160 cases, three levels in 30 cases, to exceeding three levels in 13 cases. Among these patients, 32 cases (11.76%) manifested postoperative cerebrospinal fluid (CSF) leaks (13 cases with loss of fluid from the wound and 19 cases with subcutaneous collection), necessitating careful management. Surgical revision was required in 13 instances, while resolution was achieved in 5 cases through external lumbar drainage alone, in 4 cases with a combination of surgery and subsequent external lumbar drainage, and in 10 cases through fluid aspiration coupled with compressive dressing. Notably, one patient required a blood patch due to the intricacies of dural reconstruction at the sacral level. A comparison with a cohort of 81 patients subjected to conventional sutured dural closure revealed that 19 individuals (23.46%) developed cerebrospinal fluid fistulas. Treatment modalities varied, with six cases undergoing surgical intervention, six receiving external lumbar drainage, and one requiring both surgical intervention and external lumbar drainage, while spontaneous resolution was observed in six cases.

Data were described using a number and a percentage if categorical or a mean and a standard deviation if continuous. The prevalence of a fistula in the sample was described using a number, a percentage, and a 95% confidence interval. The association with the presence of a fistula were explored with logistic regression analysis, and the results were expressed using an OR with 95% confidence interval. A significance threshold was set at 0.05. All analyses were performed with Stata version 18 (StataCorp. 2023. Stata Statistical Software: Release 18. College Station, TX, USA: StataCorp LLC).

No statistically significant correlation was found between the number of fistulas and the parameters under examination. However, an increased correlation was observed between CSF fistula occurrence and large dural openings >3 vertebrae (OR = 2.00), the lumbosacral segment (OR = 2.31), and tumor histotypes such as schwannoma (OR = 2.00), filum terminale ependymoma (OR = 2.27), and ependymoma (OR = 2.33) (Table 1).

Table 1. Statistical analysis of the correlation between CSF leak and patient data.

	All	Fistula	No Fistula	OR (95% CI)	*p*
n	272	32	240		
Sex (M)	120 (44.12%)	13 (40.62%)	107 (44.58%)	0.85 (0.40–1.80)	0.672
BMI	24.8 ± 4.4	24.4 ± 3.1	24.9 ± 4.5		
Low	13 (4.78%)	1 (3.12%)	12 (5.00%)	0.56 (0.07–4.61)	0.594
Normal	140 (51.47%)	18 (56.25%)	122 (50.83%)	1	
Over	89 (32.72%)	12 (37.50%)	77 (32.08%)	1.06 (0.48–2.31)	0.891
Obese	30 (11.03%)	1 (3.12%)	29 (12.08%)	0.23 (0.03–1.82)	0.165

Table 1. *Cont.*

	All	Fistula	No Fistula	OR (95% CI)	p
Age	55.6 ± 15.6	53.5 ± 15.5	55.9 ± 15.7	0.99 (0.97–1.01)	0.408
N involved vertebrae					
1	69 (25.37%)	9 (28.12%)	60 (25.00%)	1	
2	160 (58.82%)	17 (53.12%)	143 (59.58%)	0.79 (0.33–1.88)	0.597
3	30 (11.03%)	3 (9.38%)	27 (11.25%)	0.74 (0.19–2.95)	0.671
>3	13 (4.95%)	3 (9.38%)	10 (4.17%)	2.00 (0.46–8.68)	0.355
Spine level					
Cervical	57 (20.96%)	5 (15.62%)	52 (21.67%)	1	
Thoracic	105 (38.60%)	7 (21.88%)	98 (40.83%)	0.74 (0.22–2.46)	0.626
Lumbar-sacral	110 (40.44%)	20 (62.50%)	90 (37.50%)	2.31 (0.82–6.52)	0.114
Histology					
Meningioma	75 (27.57%)	5 (15.62%)	70 (29.17%)	1	
Schwannoma	96 (35.29%)	12 (37.50%)	84 (35.00%)	2.00 (0.67–5.95)	0.213
Ependymoma	21 (7.72%)	3 (9.38%)	18 (7.50%)	2.33 (0.51–10.69)	0.275
Ependymoma filum	43 (15.81%)	6 (18.75%)	37 (15.42%)	2.27 (0.65–7.94)	0.199
Others	37 (13.60%)	6 (18.75%)	31 (12.92%)	2.71 (0.77–9.55)	0.121

4. Discussion

Closure of the spinal dura mater following intradural tumor excision surgery poses a challenge for the surgeon due to the risk of postoperative fistula [1]. This can lead to various complications including infectious complications ranging from wound infections to meningitis, intracranial hypotension and hemorrhage, nerve root compression syndromes, and back pain [8], resulting in increased hospitalization times and costs [9]. The incidence of a fistula following intradural spinal surgery ranges from 2% to 34% [10]. Various methods and procedures for dural closure have been developed [11–13]; these may include direct suture, autologous tissue (muscle or fat), or synthetic artificial materials [3,4,14]. Additionally, reinforcement with Tachoseal® or fibrin glue can be applied [15,16].

Direct suture is the primary goal, which has a failure rate of approximately 17.5% [2]. However, as was highlighted in the systematic review by Choi et al., this failure rate is significantly reduced to a range of 5.5% to 13.7% through the adjunctive use of various materials, which decreases the incidence of CSF leak [2].

Over the years, a new dural closure method using non-penetrating metal clips [17], initially employed in vascular surgery was invented [7]. This method was first applied in pediatric and then adult spine surgeries [18,19].

Our experience involved 272 patients undergoing spinal surgery for intradural pathology where dural reconstruction was performed using the AnastoClip® Closure System (AnastoClip® Vessel Closure System, LeMaitre Vascular, Inc., Burlington, MA, USA), as is detailed in Appendix A.

Numerous investigations have examined the efficacy of these clips. Non-penetrating titanium clips offer a dural closure that exhibits immediate hydrostatic strength like intact dura, whereas suturing with either material proved notably less resilient. Moreover, the application of titanium clips demonstrated a more rapid procedure compared to suture repair [20]. Kiyoshi I. et al. conducted experimental studies comparing the hydrostatic pressure tolerance between non-penetrating titanium clips and conventional sutures. They found that the leakage pressure in the non-penetrating titanium clip group was 1.8 times higher than that in the suture group. Furthermore, the clips did not create holes, and fluid leakage occurred between them, while in the suture group, leakage occurred at the suture holes. This led them to conclude that the interrupted placement of non-penetrating titanium clips allows for dural closure without creating holes, leading to improved initial leakage pressure and reduced postoperative CSF leakage following spinal surgery [21].

Furthermore, clips suture for dural repair in a relevant animal model displayed significantly less extensive acute and chronic inflammation, foreign body reactions, and meningoneural adhesions compared to suture [22]. Studies evaluating the metallic artifacts caused by the AnastoClips® in postoperative neuroimaging have concluded that no significant alterations in evaluation quality occur postoperatively (Figure 2) [23].

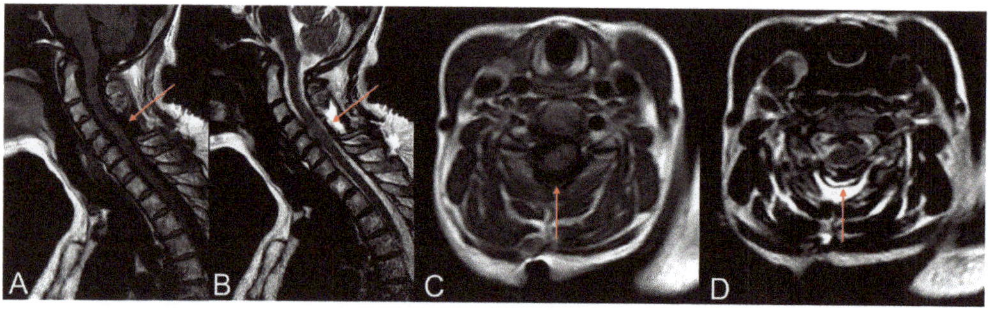

Figure 2. Titanium non-penetrating clips in the postoperative MRI (arrow). The use of clips does not compromise the quality of postoperative MRI images and does not show significant artifacts. T1 sagittal and axial plane (**A**,**C**). T2 sagittal and axial plane (**B**,**D**).

Two significant series are found in the literature, one focused on pediatric cases and the other on adults. Shane S. et al. presented a case series of 152 pediatric patients undergoing lumbar durotomy, followed by dural closure using the AnastoClip® non-penetrating titanium clip closure system. Postoperative CSF leakage occurred in 1.32% of patients at 11 and 18 days [18]. Timothy J. et al. reported on 58 patients, with a mean age of 53 years (range: 21–88), treated for spinal intradural tumors with dural closure using non-penetrating titanium clips. CSF leakage occurred in 13.7% of patients [19].

Our results confirm that the use of clips is both safe and effective in reducing the risk of CSF fistulas. Their application method is simple, operator-independent, and does not require a steep learning curve. Compared to traditional suturing, clip appliers require significantly less space for effective use, enabling a narrower surgical corridor. Clips can also be applied in closer proximity, minimizing the dead space typically created by suture threads. Additionally, the use of clips significantly reduces the time needed for dural closure, by approximately half in single-level dural openings and up to one-third in multi-level openings.

Our case series did not reveal a statistically significant correlation between postoperative fistula risk and factors such as high BMI, lumbar level, large dural openings, or specific histotypes. However, when compared to patients whose closures were performed with sutures, we observed a lower fistula rate: 11.76% with clips versus 23.46% with sutures. Notably, these results are consistent with findings reported in the adult population (11.76% vs. 13.70%).

Despite these promising outcomes, one limitation of our study is the high variability within the sample. Other limitations include the absence of randomization and the exclusion of patients who had previously undergone intradural surgery or those with dural substance loss requiring the application of dural patches.

5. Conclusions

The prevention of CSF fistulas following spinal surgery remains a significant challenge in contemporary practice. The use of non-penetrating titanium clips has been extensively documented in the literature since the early 2000s, with biomechanical studies highlighting their advantages and limitations. Based on our experience with the largest clinical series of adult patients, non-penetrating titanium clips are a safe and effective alternative to sutures, with a fistula rate of 11.76%, aligning with results reported in the literature. They reduce operative time, preserve dural integrity, and result in fewer CSF fistulas compared to traditional suturing techniques, without introducing artifacts in postoperative imaging. Their adoption could represent a significant advancement in the prevention of CSF fistulas in spinal surgery, resulting in improved patient recovery.

Author Contributions: Conceptualization, C.D.A. and L.A.; methodology, C.D.A. and L.A.; validation, C.D.A.; formal analysis, C.D.A. and L.A.; investigation, L.A., G.F., D.C. and M.C.U.; resources, C.D.A., A.O., M.T. and A.B.; data curation, L.A., G.F. and M.C.U.; writing—original draft preparation, L.A.; writing—review and editing, L.A. and C.D.A.; supervision, A.O., M.T., A.B., M.F., L.A. and C.D.A. contributed equally to this study. All authors have read and agreed to the published version of the manuscript.

Funding: This research received no external funding.

Institutional Review Board Statement: The study was conducted according to the guidelines of the Declaration of Helsinki, and approved by the Institutional Review Board (or Ethics Committee) of Humanitas Clinican and Research Hospital (protocol code 31/24 and 27/11/2024)."

Informed Consent Statement: Informed consent was obtained from all subjects involved in the study.

Data Availability Statement: Data are included in this study.

Conflicts of Interest: The authors declare no conflicts of interest.

Appendix A

Closure technique for intentional durotomy. We use the Prolene 6 0 curved needle suture thread for suspension of dura mater during dural opening and to affix two to three stiches for the closure, as is described in previously published papers on the use of titanium clips (two at the extremities of dural opening and one or two eventual stiches in the middle depending on the dural opening size) [20,21]. This approach has the advantage that the needle has the same diameter as the thread. Subsequently, we apply titanium clips for dural closure using a specialized applicator, as is described in the technical note by P. Marks et al. and the experimental studies by K. Ito et al., followed by the application of a sealant to ensure a watertight closure [17,21]. At the end, we ask the anesthetist to perform a Valsalva maneuver to check eventual tears. Finally, we close the muscular plane with detached stiches and fascial plane with tight running suture or detached stiches. The subcutaneous and cutaneous plane is performed with suture and/or staples. Usually, we use subfascial hematic for draining expect in very small openings.

Postoperative cares protocol. The subfascial drainage is removed the morning after surgery with partial mobilization for physiological function; the second day after surgery, the full mobilization is permitted. A postoperative MRI is usually performed 24 to 48 h after surgery. The hospital discharge is usually 5 to 7 days after surgery without neurological deficits. In the case of neurological deficits, the patients can be granted some days of rehabilitation in the neurosurgical ward (less than 7 days) or they can be transferred to the rehabilitation ward in our hospital or in other medical centers. If during the hospital stay, the patient develops a CSF collection, we perform, in order, (1) aspiration and compressive medication, (2) the Trendelenburg position, and (3) eventually CSF diversion by external spinal drainage. Only if all these measures fail, do we perform revision surgery. Normally, cutaneous stiches were removed 10 to 12 days after surgery. In the case of CSF collection/fistula occurring after the hospital discharge, we perform the same steps in an outpatient's regimen and in the case of persistency the patients are readmitted to the hospital and a new MRI scan is performed for decision making.

References

1. Sellin, J.N.; Kolcun, J.P.G.; Levi, A.D. Cerebrospinal Fluid Leak and Symptomatic Pseudomeningocele After Intradural Spine Surgery. *World Neurosurg.* **2018**, *120*, e497–e502. [CrossRef] [PubMed]
2. Choi, E.H.; Chan, A.Y.; Brown, N.J.; Lien, B.V.; Sahyouni, R.; Chan, A.K.; Roufail, J.; Oh, M.Y. Effectiveness of Repair Techniques for Spinal Dural Tears: A Systematic Review. *World Neurosurg.* **2021**, *149*, 140–147. [CrossRef] [PubMed]

3. Huh, J. Burr Hole Drainage: Could Be Another Treatment Option for Cerebrospinal Fluid Leakage after Unidentified Dural Tear during Spinal Surgery? *J. Korean Neurosurg. Soc.* **2013**, *53*, 59–61. [CrossRef] [PubMed]
4. Sun, X.; Sun, C.; Liu, X.; Liu, Z.; Qi, Q.; Guo, Z.; Leng, H.; Chen, Z. The frequency and treatment of dural tears and cerebrospinal fluid leakage in 266 patients with thoracic myelopathy caused by ossification of the ligamentum flavum. *Spine* **2012**, *37*, E702–E707. [CrossRef] [PubMed]
5. Robson, C.H.; Paranathala, M.P.; Dobson, G.; Ly, F.; Brown, D.P.; O'Reilly, G. Early mobilisation does not increase the complication rate from unintended lumbar durotomy. *Br. J. Neurosurg.* **2018**, *32*, 592–594. [CrossRef] [PubMed]
6. Oitment, C.; Aref, M.; Almenawar, S.; Reddy, K. Spinal Dural Repair: A Canadian Questionnaire. *Glob. Spine J.* **2018**, *8*, 359–364. [CrossRef]
7. Kirsch, W.M.; Zhu, Y.H.; Hardesty, R.A.; Chapolini, R. A new method for microvascular anastomosis: Report of experimental and clinical research. *Am. Surg.* **1992**, *58*, 722–727.
8. Takenaka, S.; Makino, T.; Sakai, Y.; Kashii, M.; Iwasaki, M.; Yoshikawa, H.; Kaito, T. Dural tear is associated with an increased rate of other perioperative complications in primary lumbar spine surgery for degenerative diseases. *Medicine* **2019**, *98*, e13970. [CrossRef]
9. Weber, C.; Piek, J.; Gunawan, D. Health care costs of incidental durotomies and postoperative cerebrospinal fluid leaks after elective spinal surgery. *Eur. Spine J.* **2015**, *24*, 2065–2068. [CrossRef]
10. Jesse, C.M.; Schermann, H.; Goldberg, J.; Gallus, M.; Häni, L.; Raabe, A.; Schär, R.T. Risk Factors for Postoperative Cerebrospinal Fluid Leakage After Intradural Spine Surgery. *World Neurosurg.* **2022**, *164*, e1190–e1199. [CrossRef]
11. Fang, Z.; Tian, R.; Jia, Y.T.; Xu, T.T.; Liu, Y. Treatment of cerebrospinal fluid leak after spine surgery. *Chin. J. Traumatol.* **2017**, *20*, 81–83. [CrossRef] [PubMed]
12. Papavero, L.; Engler, N.; Kothe, R. Incidental durotomy in spine surgery: First aid in ten steps. *Eur. Spine J.* **2015**, *24*, 2077–2084. [CrossRef] [PubMed]
13. Dong, R.P.; Zhang, Q.; Yang, L.L.; Cheng, X.L.; Zhao, J.W. Clinical management of dural defects: A review. *World J. Clin. Cases* **2023**, *11*, 2903–2915. [CrossRef] [PubMed]
14. Narotam, P.K.; José, S.; Nathoo, N.; Taylon, C.; Vora, Y. Collagen matrix (DuraGen) in dural repair: Analysis of a new modified technique. *Spine* **2004**, *29*, 2861–2869. [CrossRef]
15. Montano, N.; Pignotti, F.; Auricchio, A.M.; Fernandez, E.; Olivi, A.; Papacci, F. Results of TachoSil® associated with fibrin glue as dural sealant in a series of patients with spinal intradural tumors surgery. Technical note with a review of the literature. *J. Clin. Neurosci.* **2019**, *61*, 88–92. [CrossRef]
16. Jankowitz, B.T.; Atteberry, D.S.; Gerszten, P.C.; Karausky, P.; Cheng, B.C.; Faught, R.; Welch, W.C. Effect of fibrin glue on the prevention of persistent cerebral spinal fluid leakage after incidental durotomy during lumbar spinal surgery. *Eur. Spine J.* **2009**, *18*, 1169–1174. [CrossRef]
17. Marks, P.; Koskuba, D. Use of a non-penetrating staple device for spinal dural closure. *Br. J. Neurosurg.* **2000**, *14*, 468. [CrossRef]
18. Shahrestani, S.; Brown, N.J.; Loya, J.; Patel, N.A.; Gendreau, J.L.; Himstead, A.S.; Pierzchajlo, N.; Singh, R.; Sahyouni, R.; Diaz-Aguilar, L.D.; et al. Novel use of nonpenetrating titanium clips for pediatric primary spinal dural closure: A technical note. *Clin. Neurol. Neurosurg.* **2022**, *222*, 107422. [CrossRef]
19. Timothy, J.; Hanna, S.J.; Furtado, N.; Shanmuganathan, M.; Tyagi, A. The use of titanium non-penetrating clips to close the spinal dura. *Br. J. Neurosurg.* **2007**, *21*, 268–271. [CrossRef]
20. Faulkner, N.D.; Finn, M.A.; Anderson, P.A. Hydrostatic comparison of nonpenetrating titanium clips versus conventional suture for repair of spinal durotomies. *Spine* **2012**, *37*, E535–E539. [CrossRef]
21. Ito, K.; Aoyama, T.; Horiuchi, T.; Hongo, K. Utility of nonpenetrating titanium clips for dural closure during spinal surgery to prevent postoperative cerebrospinal fluid leakage. *J. Neurosurg. Spine* **2015**, *23*, 812–819. [CrossRef] [PubMed]
22. Palm, S.J.; Kirsch, W.M.; Zhu, Y.H.; Peckham, N.; Kihara, S.-I.; Anton, R.; Anton, T.; Balzer, K.; Eickmann, T. Dural closure with nonpenetrating clips prevents meningoneural adhesions: An experimental study in dogs. *Neurosurgery* **1999**, *45*, 875–882. [CrossRef] [PubMed]
23. Ito, K.; Seguchi, T.; Nakamura, T.; Chiba, A.; Hasegawa, T.; Nagm, A.; Horiuchi, T.; Hongo, K. Evaluation of Metallic Artifacts Caused by Nonpenetrating Titanium Clips in Postoperative Neuroimaging. *World Neurosurg.* **2016**, *96*, 16–22. [CrossRef] [PubMed]

brain sciences

MDPI

Article

High Accuracy of Three-Dimensional Navigated Kirschner-Wire-Less Single-Step Pedicle Screw System (SSPSS) in Lumbar Fusions: Comparison of Intraoperatively Planned versus Final Screw Position

Mateusz Bielecki, Blake I. Boadi, Yizhou Xie, Chibuikem A. Ikwuegbuenyi, Minaam Farooq, Jessica Berger, Alan Hernández-Hernández, Ibrahim Hussain and Roger Härtl *

Weill Cornell Medicine—Department of Neurosurgery, NewYork-Presbyterian Och Spine Hospital, New York, NY 10034, USA; drahh9208@gmail.com (A.H.-H.)

* Correspondence: roh9005@med.cornell.edu

Abstract: (1) Background: Our team has previously introduced the Single-Step Pedicle Screw System (SSPSS), which eliminates the need for K-wires, as a safe and effective method for percutaneous minimally invasive spine (MIS) pedicle screw placement. Despite this, there are ongoing concerns about the reliability and accuracy of screw placement in MIS procedures without traditional tools like K-wires and Jamshidi needles. To address these concerns, we evaluated the accuracy of the SSPSS workflow by comparing the planned intraoperative screw trajectories with the final screw positions. Traditionally, screw placement accuracy has been assessed by grading the final screw position using postoperative CT scans. (2) Methods: We conducted a retrospective review of patients who underwent lumbar interbody fusion, using intraoperative 3D navigation for screw placement. The planned screw trajectories were saved in the navigation system during each procedure, and postoperative CT scans were used to evaluate the implanted screws. Accuracy was assessed by comparing the Gertzbein and Robbins classification scores of the planned trajectories and the final screw positions. Accuracy was defined as a final screw position matching the classification of the planned trajectory. (3) Results: Out of 206 screws, 196 (95%) were accurately placed, with no recorded complications. (4) Conclusions: The SSPSS workflow, even without K-wires and other traditional instruments, facilitates accurate and reliable pedicle screw placement.

Keywords: accuracy; minimally invasive; screw placement; navigation; 3D-NAV; pedicle screw; SSPSS; MIS; MISS

1. Introduction

With accurate and safe screw placement, short- and long-term complications such as the penetrance of the spinal canal or adjacent vessels, pseudoarthrosis, adjacent segment disease, and neural injury or irritation can be avoided [1–3]. Many surgeons have used intraoperative navigation for screw placement to ensure precision. Navigation provides remarkable soft-tissue and bone imaging quality that is superior to fluoroscopy [4,5].

Pedicle screw placement has traditionally required pedicle probing instruments such as Kirschner wires (K-wires) and Jamshidi needles. Some surgeons believe that such instruments are absolutely necessary for accurate and reproducible placement of pedicle screws. Our group, however, implemented an advanced spinal fusion technique, known as the navigated Single-Step Pedicle Screw System (SSPSS), in which the use of K-wires was eliminated for percutaneous pedicle screw insertion. Instead of a K-wire or Jamshidi needle, a navigated stylet was incorporated at the tip of the navigated screw inserter which allowed for docking on the superior articulating facet of the indicated level. This was followed by screw insertion over the stylet [6].

The navigated SSPSS workflow tackles many of the challenges associated with conventional pedicle screw placement. Vertebral anatomy varies across patients, and with navigation, surgeons can meticulously plan a screw trajectory and localize the preferred region to be instrumented efficiently. Without navigation, surgeons are required to consistently verify anatomy with fluoroscopy which can prolong a procedure. Jamshidi needles and K-wires are also tedious to work with and can cause nerve damage or vascular injury [7,8]. With docking, tapping, and screw insertion combined into one seamless procedure with the SSPSS device, the repetitive and laborious process of various instrument use and fluoroscopic confirmation is eliminated.

In our recently published study, the "totally navigated" SSPSS workflow produced a 90% grade 0 breach [5,6]. When we assessed the accuracy of implanted screws in our previously published study, we only assessed anatomical accuracy postoperatively with CT scans, as much of the existing literature has. We subsequently sought a more detailed approach to assessment and decided to compare planned intraoperative screw trajectories with final screw position using the Gertzbein and Robbins classification system [9]. A comparison between intended pedicle screw placement and final screw position offers surgeons a better evaluation of how closely their surgical execution matches their planning. If there are any major deviations between intended and final screw position, surgeons can study these errors and devise plans to avoid them in the future. Given our previously reported 90% grade 0 breach, we anticipated a high percentage of screws placed exactly as intraoperatively planned.

2. Materials and Methods

2.1. Patient Information

This study was a retrospective single-center study focused on consecutive patients receiving instrumented fusion for lumbar degenerative disc disease. Indications for surgery included spondylolisthesis with or without neurogenic claudication, foraminal stenosis, or facet arthropathy with degenerative dynamic instability. Figure 1 shows a sample case. Patients were included from January 2022 until August 2022. Those included were over 18 years of age and underwent a transforaminal lumbar interbody fusion (TLIF), anterior lumbar interbody fusion (ALIF), or lateral lumbar interbody fusion (LLIF) procedure with the navigable SSPSS workflow. Patients with previous lumbar spinal surgery, osteoporosis, and spine fractures were excluded. Informed consent was obtained from all included patients.

2.2. Surgical Approach

Following general endotracheal anesthesia set-up and neurophysiologic monitoring needles, patients were positioned in the prone position. Intraoperative electromyography (EMG) monitoring was operated by a neurophysiology specialist throughout the procedure to avoid nerve injury. Excess skin and fat were taped down. The Brainlab (Brainlab AG, Munich, Germany) reference array was then fixed into the iliac crest using Steinmann pins. An intraoperative CT scan was performed and registered with navigation software. A pedicle screw trajectory was subsequently planned and graded with the 3D navigation system wand and stored for subsequent analysis. The SSPSS device with navigation star was registered and calibrated after the navigation wand was used to identify the desired trajectory (Figure 2). A stylet at the tip of the screw insertion device was used to dock on the aspect of the superior articulating facet of the level to be engaged both ipsilaterally and contralaterally. With this stylet, the surgeon was able eliminate K-wires and other risky pedicle-probing instruments from the surgical workflow. With gentle malleting, the stylet was inserted in the bone, and the screw was fully engaged into the pedicle. Once the pedicle screw was safely inserted into the pedicle, the device with the stylet attached was retracted. All screws used were Viper Prime System Screws (DePuy Spine, Raynham, MA, USA). As cited in our previous study, the navigated SSPSS workflow can be briefly summarized in the following steps:

1. A skin incision is marked using navigation guidance.
2. Navigation is manually verified using the Brainlab pointer to identify and palate a transverse process at a distance from the reference array.
3. The navigated screw with the screw driver is calibrated.
4. After inserting the screw, the screws are test stimulated with an extended electrode probe. A threshold of 8 mA is used to consider screw repositioning.
5. A final intraoperative CT is completed with the navigation reference in place in case of further instrument adjustment or decompression.
6. The patient's wound is generously irrigated and washed after meticulous hemostasis is performed. Osteo-stimulative bone graft is packed under the rod. Local anesthesia is used to infiltrate the muscle and the wound is closed [6].

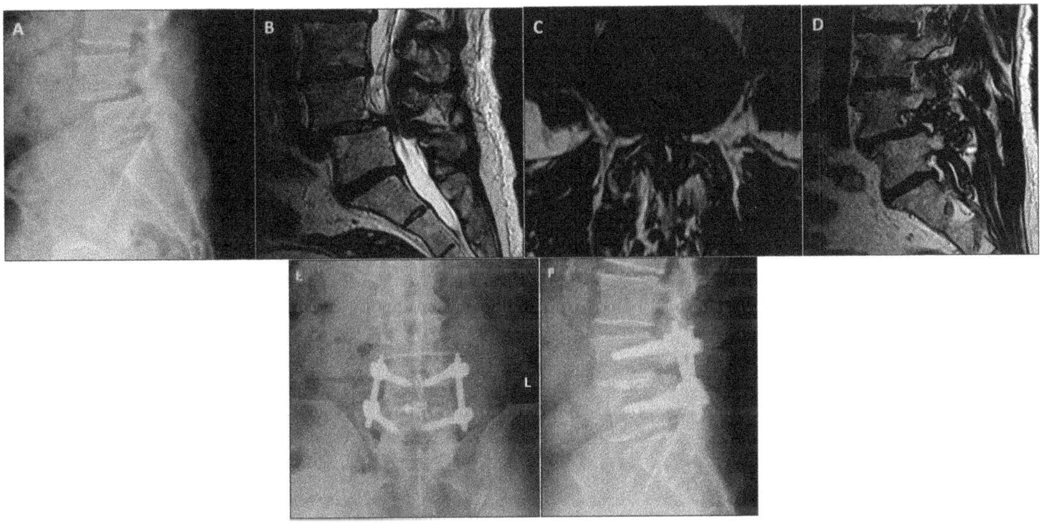

Figure 1. Imaging studies of a patient with degenerative spondylolisthesis who underwent minimally invasive TLIF and pedicle screw placement using the SPSS. (**A**) Lateral X-ray demonstrating L4/5 spondylolisthesis. (**B**) Sagittal MRI illustrating the left L4/5 foramen. (**C**) Axial MRI of the L4/5 level shows narrowing of the lumbar spinal canal. (**D**) Sagittal MRI illustrating the right L4/5 foramen. (**E**) Coronal postoperative radiograph after L4/5 minimally invasive TLIF. (**F**) Sagittal postoperative radiograph after L4/5 minimally invasive TLIF.

2.3. *Analysis*

General patient data collected included patient age, sex, and surgical specific outcomes including fusion technique, levels fused, revisions, and complications. Planned screw trajectories were compared with final screw placement based on the Gertzbein and Robbins grading system (Figure 3) [9]. This classification system requires the user to grade the anatomical placement of a screw ranging from grade A, meaning fully within the pedicle without any breaches to grade E, demonstrating a breach outside of the pedicle cortex by more than 6 mm (Figure 4). The complete grading system described by Gertzbein and Robbins is as follows: Grade A: screw completely within the pedicle, Grade B: screw breaches the pedicle cortex by less than 2 mm, Grade C: screw breaches pedicle cortex by less than 4 mm, Grade D: screw breaches pedicle cortex by less than 6 mm, Grade E: screw breaches pedicle by greater than 6 mm [9]. Breaches can be cranial, lateral, medial, or caudal (Figure 4). Screw trajectories were measured intraoperatively using Brainlab software, and images and measurements were stored. Final screw insertion was graded on postoperative CT scans using the Vue Motion PACS system. Accuracy was defined as a screw that had the same classification when compared to the intraoperative planned screw

(Figure 5). Grade discrepancies with breaches between planned and final screw position were considered misplaced screws. Screw placement was graded by two fellowship-trained spine surgeons independently and disagreements were resolved by discussion. All other relevant clinical and operative information were collected from electronic medical records.

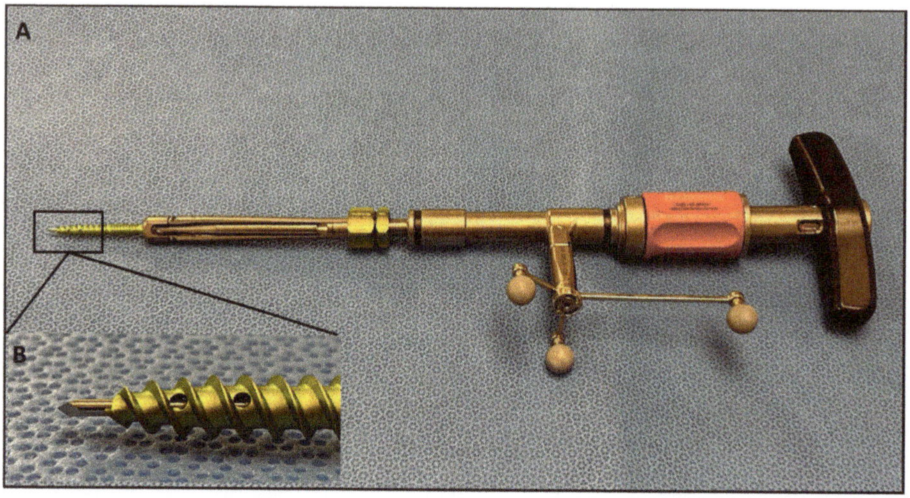

Figure 2. (**A**) SSPSS navigated screw inserter with spheres attached, forming the navigation star. The navigation star is crucial for navigation registration and intraoperative anatomical localization. (**B**) Close-up view of the screw inserter showing the navigated stylet.

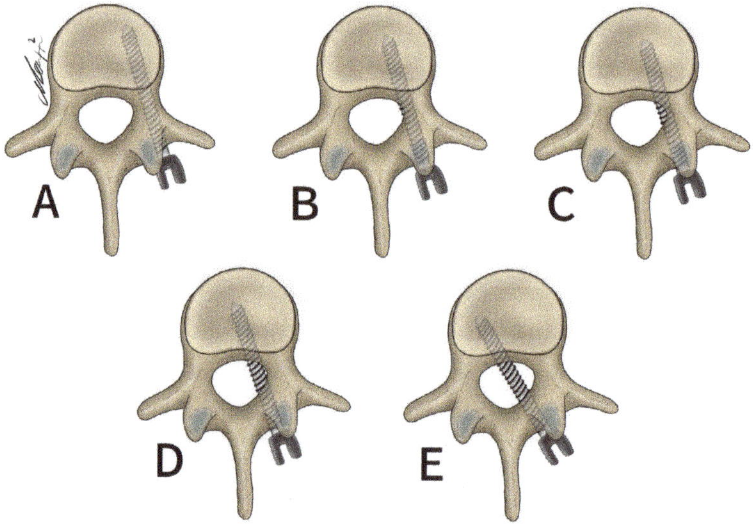

Figure 3. Gertzbein and Robbins classification system. (**A**) 0 mm breach. (**B**) <2 mm breach. (**C**) <4 mm breach. (**D**) <6 mm breach. (**E**) >6 mm breach.

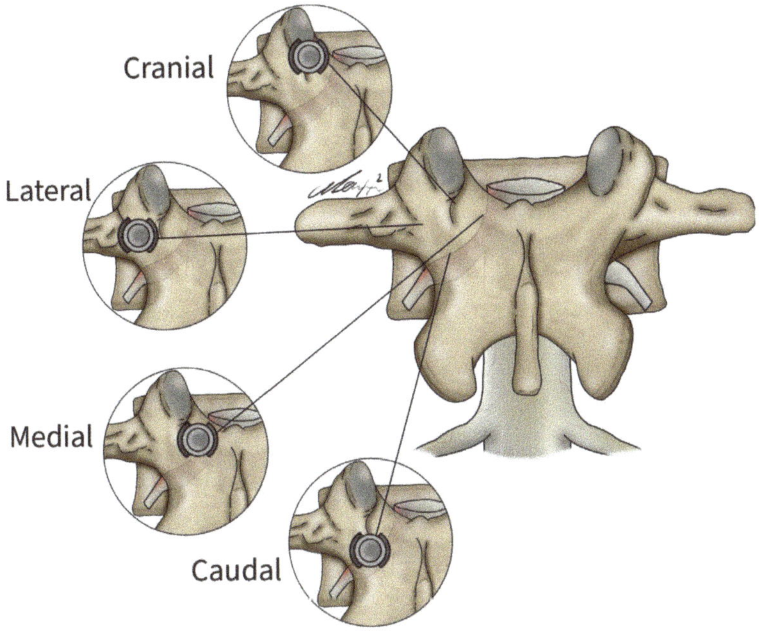

Figure 4. Lateral, medial, cranial, and caudal screw breaches demonstrated within the vertebral body.

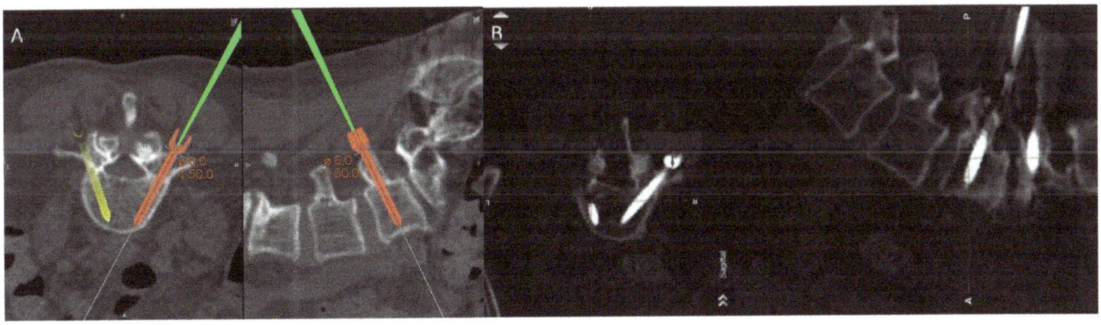

Figure 5. Percutaneous pedicle screw insertion intraoperative imaging. (**A**) Grade A screw trajectory planned at the right L5 with navigation wand. (**B**) Final pedicle screw inserted within planned Grade A trajectory at the right L5 pedicle.

3. Results

3.1. Patient and Surgery Characteristics

Between January and August 2022, 47 patients with lumbar interbody fusions were included in this analysis. Table 1 provides an overview of patient and surgery characteristics. The mean age of the cohort was 64.1 ± 13.3 years. A total of 24 (51.1%) were male. The mean BMI was 27.6 ± 5.1. Of all patients, 38 (80.9%) underwent a TLIF, and 5 (10.6%) underwent an XLIF, while the remaining 4 patients received an ALIF (2, 4.3%) and a PLIF (2, 4.3%). A total of 38 patients (80.9%) were fused at one level, 7 (14.9%) at two levels, and 2 (4.3%) at three levels. Spinal stenosis was the most prevalent diagnosis, affecting 34% of patients, followed by lumbar radiculopathy (23.4%) and spondylolisthesis (19.1%). Intraoperative blood loss was typically low, with 27.7% of patients losing less than 50 mL and 48.9% losing between 50 and 150 mL. The median duration of surgery was

182 min (IQR: 144–225), and the median hospital stay was 48 h (IQR: 24–108). There were no intraoperative or immediate postoperative reported complications in this cohort.

Table 1. Patient and surgery characteristics.

Characteristic	Frequency (n = 47)
Age (years)	64.1 ± 13.3
Sex	
Male	24 (51.1%)
Female	23 (49.9%)
BMI (kg/m^2)	27.6 ± 5.1
Fusion technique	
ALIF	2 (4.3%)
PLIF	2 (4.3%)
TLIF	38 (80.9%)
XLIF	5 (10.6%)
Number of levels fused	
1	38 (80.9%)
2	7 (14.9%)
3	2 (4.3%)
Primary Diagnosis	
Spinal stenosis	16 (34)
Lumbar radiculopathy	11 (23.4)
Spondylolisthesis	9 (19.1)
DDD	6 (12.8)
Others	5 (10.6)
Revision during follow-up	2 (4.3%)
Adjacent segment disease	2
Blood Loss (n, %)	
<50 mL	13 (27.7)
50–150 mL	23 (48.9)
>150 mL	11 (23.4)
Duration of surgery (minutes), median (IQR)	182 (144–225)
Length of hospital stay (hours), median (IQR)	48 (24–108)

DDD, degenerative disc disease; Others (revision, revision and extension, spondylosis, closed unstable burst fracture).

3.2. Screw Placement and Accuracy

Table 2 provides an overview of the number of screws per vertebral body. All levels operated received bilateral screws. In total, 206 screws were placed with 103 on both the right and left side. Most screws were placed at L5 (84 screws) followed by L4 (68 screws). A total of 2 screws were placed at L1, 4 at L2, 20 at L3, and 28 at S1. In total, 10 screws (4.9%) placed were classified as breaches. These screws were placed at L4 on the left side (four screws), L4 on the right side (two screws), L5 on the left side (three screws), and S1 on the right side (one screw). Table 3 demonstrates how the intended placement of these screws deviated from their final location according to the Gertzbein and Robbins classification. Eight screws were planned as "A" but were placed as a "B". One screw was perioperatively planned as "A" and was placed as a "C". Finally, one screw was planned as a "B" and was placed as an "A". In total, 196/206 (95%) screws were placed accurately.

Table 2. Number of screws inserted per vertebral levels.

Vertebral Body	Screw Position		Total
	Right	Left	
L1	1	1	2
L2	2	2	4
L3	10	10	20
L4	34 (2) *	34 (4) *	68
L5	42	42 (3) *	84
S1	14 (1) *	14	28
Total	103	103	206

* Number of screws that changed from the planned position.

Table 3. Comparison between intraoperatively planned screws and final screw position using the Gertzbein and Robbins classification system.

		Inserted Screws			
		A	B	C	Total
Planned	A	195	8	1	204
	B	1	1	0	2
	C	0	0	0	0
	Total	196	9	1	206

4. Discussion

We sought to assess the accuracy of the SSPSS workflow for screw placement in the lumbar spine based on comparisons between intended/planned screw placement and the final location of the screw following placement. Previous studies have focused primarily on the anatomical accuracy of screw placement and screw breach evasion using only postoperative imaging. With the use of a navigation system, we were able to store our intraoperatively planned screw trajectories and compare these trajectories to CT imaging of the implanted screw. A total of 95% of pedicle screws inserted were inserted as "A". Some screws intraoperatively planned as "grade B" were inserted as "grade A". Such placement would not be defined as accurate with our definition. However, these screws were still implanted completely within the pedicle.

The impetus for our described SSPSS workflow was eliminating tedious traditional MIS methods and instrumentation such as K-wires. The use of K-wires carries risk. They can bend, causing difficulty with the passage of cannulated instruments over them. They can also penetrate the vertebral body, usually in osteoporotic patients, causing vascular or visceral injury or migrating into the spinal canal and causing infection. These complications can increase patient morbidity, operative time, radiation exposure, and surgeon frustration [10–12]. The navigated SSPSS workflow also addresses variations in patient anatomy that make screw placement difficult. With preoperative planning, surgeons can study patient anatomy in high detail and choose the best screws and implants for each patient. Intraoperatively, surgeons can also observe patient anatomy in real time. This starkly contrasts with repetitive fluoroscopy shots for anatomical understanding and localization. Spine surgeons can be actively engaged throughout the procedure without interruption with real-time navigation. Repetitive cannulation in multiple steps is also required for conventional screw placement. The literature has shown that the traditional, non-navigated method for the placement of pedicle screws is more likely to require intraoperative correction when compared to navigated screws. With intraoperative CT, poorly placed screws can be identified and re-positioned before the conclusion of the operation. This diminishes the need for revision surgeries. A human cadaver study confirmed that CT improved pedicle screw placement accuracy by up to 87%. [13] A meta-analysis found that out of 8539 screws placed, the perforation risk for navigation was 6% compared to 15% for free-hand placement without CT [14]. As the accuracy of screw placement increases with the assistance of intraoperative CT, the amount of radiation delivered to surgical staff also decreases [14–16]. With the navigated SSPSS system, pedicle screw placement becomes seamless. Docking, malleting, and screw insertion become integrated into a continuous routine, reducing unnecessary mental and physical demands on the surgeon.

No revision surgeries and neurologic or vascular complications were reported in our first described use of the SSPSS workflow, which led us to conclude that outcomes of fusions with the technique are favorable and traditional instrumentation like K-wires are not necessary for safety and accuracy [6]. In this study, we report a high accuracy of screws placed as planned with the same SSPSS workflow, once again demonstrating no need for stand-alone K-wires, Jamshidi needles, or other pedicle probing instruments in fusions for lumbar degenerative disc disease. Additionally, we observed that intraoperative blood loss was low, with 48.9% losing between 50 and 150 mL, and the mean surgical time was 182 min. These results demonstrate the efficiency and effectiveness of the SSPSS. The streamlined nature of this system likely contributed to reduced intraoperative bleeding and shorter surgical times compared to traditional multi-step systems.

While the SSPSS workflow does incorporate a navigated stylet that does serve somewhat of a similar function to the K-wire, its small size and ease of use make the stylet quite different and superior. With a navigation system, the surgeon can easily monitor the style in real time as it is docked and engaged into the patient's bone. This greatly reduces the risk of visceral and vascular injury or unintended migration that K-wires pose. The navigation system we used also undoubtedly accounted for the high accuracy we observed between intraoperatively planned and postoperative screws. Previous studies have confirmed that non-navigated screws were more likely to require intraoperative correction than navigated screws [6].

Miller et al. assessed the accuracy of implanted pedicle screws in the thoracic and lumbosacral spine based on a planned trajectory [17]. Of 240 screws placed, the mean angular difference between the planned trajectory and implanted screw was $2.17^\circ \pm 2.20^\circ$ on axial images and $2.16^\circ \pm 2.24^\circ$ on sagittal images. These angular differences are small and are comparable to the high placement accuracy we achieved in our study. Ganguly et al. also reviewed the difference between 59 planned and postprocedural pedicle screw locations and observed a small mean difference of 2.8 mm; however, K-wires were used in this study [18]. To our knowledge, this is the first study to compare intraoperatively planned screw positions with final placements in evaluating pedicle screw placement accuracy using the SPSS workflow without K-wires [19–22].

Fujita et al. reconstructed a 3D model from pre-operative CT data using MySpine® system (accessible via the MySpine web planner). They designed a pre-operative surgical plan for pedicle screw placement which included screw diameter, length, and direction in transverse and sagittal angles. Using this model as a guide, pedicle screws were placed. The authors then compared the 3D models with postoperative CT scans. Of all previous studies reviewed, this method of screw accuracy assessment is most similar to ours. However, there are differences. With the use of the Brainlab navigation system, we were able to plan and place pedicle screws during the operation. Fujita et al. planned pedicle screw insertion preoperatively. Fujita et al. also compared planned and final screw positions with angular deviations, while our study used the Gertzbein and Robbins grading system to evaluate differences. An important similarity between both studies is the patient-specific pedicle screw planning afforded by both the MySpine (accessible via the MySpine web planner) and Brainlab systems (Munich, Germany) [23].

A surgical challenge of utilizing SSPSS is the potential for motion changes by surgeons during pedicle screw insertion to impact the recognition of intraoperative imaging. One scenario where we often encounter an intraoperative change in screw trajectory, differing from the preoperative plan, is when there is skiving of the stylet extending out of the SPSS due to a steep angle at the SAP/transverse process junction. In such cases, the screw may deviate laterally and fail to capture the pedicle. To overcome this challenge, we identify a new starting point that does not match the preplanned trajectory and adjust the trajectory to maximize pedicle capture. We use a navigated awl-tip tap, which has a sharper tip and can either follow the initial starting point or establish a new one. If this method is ineffective, we use the new starting point with the stylet. These adjustments help ensure accurate screw placement despite the challenges posed by intraoperative motion.

This study is not without its limitations. First, we recognize that the sample size for our study is small. As we continue to use the SSPSS workflow in lumbar fusions, we will continue to assess the accuracy of the technique with technological advancements like AR and robotics in more patients. Second, the single-arm design does not include a comparative analysis with the conventional free-hand technique. This limits our ability to definitively conclude that the observed benefits are superior to those achieved with traditional methods. Future studies should incorporate comparative, randomized controlled trials to provide a more robust assessment of the efficacy and advantages of the single-step pedicle screw system over conventional techniques. Third, we only used one method for accuracy assessment. We believe, however, that our use of the Gertzbein and Robbins grading system is a valid and reliable method to assess accuracy. However, we acknowledge the intrinsic differences in screw classification. Specifically, deviation from the initial plan should consider the entry point, the tip of the screw, and angulation rather than simply differentiating between GRS A, B, and C screws. While we focused on GRS due to its clinical significance and widespread acceptance, we recognize that future studies assessing accuracy should incorporate more precise measurements of screw placement accuracy. This includes evaluating deviations in the entry point, the tip of the screw, and angulation. Additionally, considering the ratio of pedicle diameter to screw diameter is crucial for a comprehensive assessment. Future research comparing intraoperative trajectory planning and postoperative imaging with the SSPSS workflow should therefore expand beyond classification systems like GRS and include numerical deviations for a more precise evaluation of screw placement accuracy.

5. Conclusions

Overall, our study demonstrates a high accuracy of pedicle screw placement when compared with intraoperatively planned trajectories for lumbar interbody fusions. K-wires and other traditional pedicle probing instruments are not needed for the accurate implantation of pedicle screws if the SSPSS workflow is employed.

Author Contributions: Conceptualization, I.H. and R.H.; methodology, M.B., B.I.B., Y.X., I.H. and R.H.; software, I.H. and R.H.; validation, I.H. and R.H.; formal analysis, M.B., Y.X. and C.A.I.; investigation, M.B., B.I.B., Y.X., I.H. and R.H.; resources, R.H.; data curation, B.I.B. and J.B.; writing—original draft preparation, M.B., B.I.B., Y.X. and I.H.; writing—review and editing, M.B., B.I.B., Y.X., C.A.I., M.F., J.B., A.H.-H., I.H. and R.H.; visualization, A.H.-H.; supervision, I.H. and R.H.; project administration, I.H. and R.H.; funding acquisition, R.H. All authors have read and agreed to the published version of the manuscript.

Funding: This research received no external funding.

Institutional Review Board Statement: This study was performed in accordance with the ethical standards of the Declaration of Helsinki (as revised in 2013) and was approved by the Weill Cornell Medicine (WCM) Institutional Review Board (IRB) (approval number: 1912021199) and individual consent for this retrospective analysis was waived.

Informed Consent Statement: Patient consent was waived due to the retrospective nature of this study. The extracted data included clinical data only and did not include any personally identifiable information. Therefore, the need for informed consent was waived.

Data Availability Statement: The data presented here are available upon request from the corresponding author. They are not publicly available because of ethical concerns.

Conflicts of Interest: Roger Hartl declares consulting work for DePuy Synthes, Brainlab, and Ulrich. Roger Hartl reports a financial relationship with Zimmer Biomet and Real Spine. No other author declares any financial interests or personal relationships.

References

1. Laine, T.; Mäkitalo, K.; Schlenzka, D.; Tallroth, K.; Poussa, M.; Alho, A. Accuracy of Pedicle Screw Insertion: A Prospective CT Study in 30 Low Back Patients. *Eur. Spine J.* **1997**, *6*, 402–405. [CrossRef]
2. Verma, R.; Krishan, S.; Haendlmayer, K.; Mohsen, A. Functional Outcome of Computer-Assisted Spinal Pedicle Screw Placement: A Systematic Review and Meta-Analysis of 23 Studies Including 5,992 Pedicle Screws. *Eur. Spine J.* **2010**, *19*, 370–375. [CrossRef] [PubMed]
3. Ahmadian, A.; Deukmedjian, A.R.; Abel, N.; Dakwar, E.; Uribe, J.S. Analysis of Lumbar Plexopathies and Nerve Injury after Lateral Retroperitoneal Transpsoas Approach: Diagnostic Standardization. *J. Neurosurg. Spine* **2013**, *18*, 289–297. [CrossRef]
4. Goldstein, C.L.; Macwan, K.; Sundararajan, K.; Rampersaud, Y.R. Comparative Outcomes of minimally Invasive Surgery for Posterior Lumbar Fusion: A Systematic Review. *Clin. Orthop. Relat. Res.* **2014**, *472*, 1727–1737. [CrossRef] [PubMed]
5. Lian, X.; Navarro-Ramirez, R.; Berlin, C.; Jada, A.; Moriguchi, Y.; Zhang, Q.; Härtl, R. Total 3D Airo® Navigation for minimally Invasive Transforaminal Lumbar Interbody Fusion. *Biomed. Res. Int.* **2016**, *2016*, 5027340. [CrossRef] [PubMed]
6. Schmidt, F.A.; Lekuya, H.M.; Kirnaz, S.; Hernandez, R.N.; Hussain, I.; Chang, L.; Navarro-Ramirez, R.; Wipplinger, C.; Rawanduzy, C.; Härtl, R. Novel MIS 3D NAV Single Step Pedicle Screw System (SSPSS): Workflow, Accuracy and Initial Clinical Experience. *Global Spine J.* **2022**, *12*, 1098–1108. [CrossRef] [PubMed]
7. Scheer, J.K.; Harvey, M.J.; Dahdaleh, N.S.; Smith, Z.A.; Fessler, R.G. K-Wire Fracture during minimally Invasive Transforaminal Lumbar Interbody Fusion: Report of Six Cases and Recommendations for Avoidance and Management. *Surg. Neurol. Int.* **2014**, *5*, S520–S522. [CrossRef]
8. Peterson, A.; Ngai, L.K.; Burbridge, M.A. Intraoperative Kirschner Wire Migration during Robotic minimally Invasive Spine Surgery. *Case Rep. Anesthesiol.* **2019**, *2019*, 9581285. [CrossRef]
9. Gertzbein, S.D.; Robbin, S.E. Accuracy of Pedicular Screw Placement In Vivo. *Spine (Phila. Pa. 1976)* **1990**, *15*, 11–14. [CrossRef]
10. Minić, L.; Lepić, M.; Novaković, N.; Mandić-Rajčević, S. Symptomatic Migration of a Kirschner Wire into the Spinal Canal without Spinal Cord Injury: Case Report. *J. Neurosurg. Spine* **2016**, *24*, 291–294. [CrossRef]
11. Spitz, S.M.; Sandhu, F.A.; Voyadzis, J.-M. Percutaneous "K-Wireless" Pedicle Screw Fixation Technique: An Evaluation of the Initial Experience of 100 Screws with Assessment of Accuracy, Radiation Exposure, and Procedure Time. *J. Neurosurg. Spine* **2015**, *22*, 422–431. [CrossRef] [PubMed]
12. Mobbs, R.J.; Raley, D.A. Complications with K-Wire Insertion for Percutaneous Pedicle Screws. *J. Spinal Disord. Tech.* **2014**, *27*, 390–394. [CrossRef] [PubMed]
13. Learch, T.J.; Massie, J.B.; Pathria, M.N.; Ahlgren, B.A.; Garfin, S.R. Assessment of Pedicle Screw Placement Utilizing Conventional Radiography and Computed Tomography: A Proposed Systematic Approach to Improve Accuracy of Interpretation. *Spine (Phila. Pa. 1976)* **2004**, *29*, 767–773. [CrossRef]
14. Shin, B.J.; James, A.R.; Njoku, I.U.; Härtl, R. Pedicle Screw Navigation: A Systematic Review and Meta-Analysis of Perforation Risk for Computer-Navigated versus Freehand Insertion. *J. Neurosurg. Spine* **2012**, *17*, 113–122. [CrossRef]
15. Ughwanogho, E.; Patel, N.M.; Baldwin, K.D.; Sampson, N.R.; Flynn, J.M. Computed Tomography-Guided Navigation of Thoracic Pedicle Screws for Adolescent Idiopathic Scoliosis Results in More Accurate Placement and Less Screw Removal. *Spine (Phila. Pa. 1976)* **2012**, *37*, E473–E478. [CrossRef]
16. Härtl, R.; Lam, K.S.; Wang, J.; Korge, A.; Kandziora, F.; Audigé, L. Worldwide Survey on the Use of Navigation in Spine Surgery. *World Neurosurg.* **2013**, *79*, 162–172. [CrossRef]
17. Miller, C.A.; Ledonio, C.G.; Hunt, M.A.; Siddiq, F.; Polly, D.W. Reliability of the Planned Pedicle Screw Trajectory versus the Actual Pedicle Screw Trajectory Using Intra-Operative 3D CT and Image Guidance. *Int. J. Spine Surg.* **2016**, *10*, 38. [CrossRef]
18. Ganguly, R.; minnema, A.; Singh, V.; Grossbach, A. Retrospective Analysis of Pedicle Screw Accuracy for Patients Undergoing Spinal Surgery Assisted by Intraoperative Computed Tomography (CT) Scanner AIRO® and BrainLab© Navigation. *Clin. Neurol. Neurosurg.* **2020**, *198*, 106113. [CrossRef] [PubMed]
19. Molina, C.A.; Sciubba, D.M.; Greenberg, J.K.; Khan, M.; Witham, T. Clinical Accuracy, Technical Precision, and Workflow of the First in Human Use of an Augmented-Reality Head-Mounted Display Stereotactic Navigation System for Spine Surgery. *Oper. Neurosurg.* **2021**, *20*, 300–309. [CrossRef]
20. Oertel, M.F.; Hobart, J.; Stein, M.; Schreiber, V.; Scharbrodt, W. Clinical and Methodological Precision of Spinal Navigation Assisted by 3D Intraoperative O-Arm Radiographic Imaging. *J. Neurosurg. Spine* **2011**, *14*, 532–536. [CrossRef]
21. Molina, C.A.; Phillips, F.M.; Colman, M.W.; Ray, W.Z.; Khan, M.; Orru', E.; Poelstra, K.; Khoo, L. A Cadaveric Precision and Accuracy Analysis of Augmented Reality-Mediated Percutaneous Pedicle Implant Insertion. *J. Neurosurg. Spine* **2020**, *34*, 316–324. [CrossRef] [PubMed]
22. Gubian, A.; Kausch, L.; Neumann, J.-O.; Kiening, K.; Ishak, B.; Maier-Hein, K.; Unterberg, A.; Scherer, M. CT-Navigated Spinal Instrumentations-Three-Dimensional Evaluation of Screw Placement Accuracy in Relation to a Screw Trajectory Plan. *Medicina* **2022**, *58*, 1200. [CrossRef] [PubMed]

23. Fujita, R.; Oda, I.; Takeuchi, H.; Oshima, S.; Fujiya, M.; Yahara, Y.; Kawaguchi, Y. Accuracy of Pedicle Screw Placement Using Patient-Specific Template Guide System. *J. Orthop. Sci.* **2022**, *27*, 348–354. [CrossRef] [PubMed]

brain sciences

MDPI

Article

Flow Diversion for Cerebral Aneurysms: A Decade-Long Experience with Improved Outcomes and Predictors of Success

Tae Keun Jee [1], Je Young Yeon [1], Keon Ha Kim [2], Jong-Soo Kim [1] and Pyoung Jeon [2,*]

1 Department of Neurosurgery, Samsung Medical Center, Sungkyunkwan University School of Medicine, Seoul 06351, Republic of Korea; taekeun.jee@samsung.com (T.K.J.); yeonjay.youn@samsung.com (J.Y.Y.)
2 Department of Radiology, Samsung Medical Center, Sungkyunkwan University School of Medicine, Seoul 06351, Republic of Korea
* Correspondence: drpjeon@gmail.com; Tel.: +82-2-3410-6433; Fax: +82-2-3410-0048

Abstract: Background: Flow diversion has significantly improved the management of cerebral aneurysms. Technological advancements and increased clinical experience over the past decade have led to better outcomes and fewer complications. This study provides updated results and examines the factors that influence the success of flow diversion. Methods: We reviewed records of 115 patients with 121 intracranial aneurysms treated from July 2014 to August 2023. All patients had unruptured aneurysms in the anterior and posterior circulation. Results: Complete aneurysm occlusion was achieved in 72.7% of cases, with a complication rate of 9.1%. Significant predictors of complete occlusion included aneurysm diameter (OR = 0.89, 95% CI 0.82–0.97, $p = 0.009$) and the presence of incorporated branches (OR = 0.22, 95% CI 0.08–0.59, $p = 0.003$). Cox analysis identified neck diameter (HR = 0.92, 95% CI 0.87–0.98, $p = 0.009$) and incorporated branch (HR = 0.40, 95% CI 0.24–0.69, $p = 0.001$) as significant for occlusion. Multivariable analysis identified aneurysm diameter (OR = 1.21, 95% CI 1.09–1.37, $p = 0.001$) as significant for safety outcomes. Improved outcomes were observed in recent treatments, with higher occlusion rates (79.7% vs. 61.7%, $p = 0.050$) and lower complication rates (4.1% vs. 14.9%, $p = 0.011$). Conclusions: Enhanced technical proficiency, better devices, and refined patient selection have significantly improved the efficacy and safety of flow diversion for cerebral aneurysms. Identifying significant predictors for treatment success and safety outcomes can inform clinical practice, aiding in patient selection.

Keywords: flow diversion; cerebral aneurysm; aneurysm occlusion; long-term outcomes; safety outcomes

1. Introduction

Flow diversion stents have revolutionized the treatment of cerebral aneurysms, particularly those that are difficult to manage with traditional methods [1,2]. These stents redirect blood flow away from the aneurysm, promoting thrombosis and eventual occlusion. Numerous studies have been conducted on flow diversion, with early research highlighting its promising outcomes and subsequent studies providing evidence on when flow diversion is more advantageous [3–6]. Understanding the specific characteristics and outcomes associated with flow diversion is essential for improving the overall treatment results. When unfavorable outcomes occur after flow diversion, subsequent treatment options are significantly limited, often constrained to either deploying additional flow diverters or performing parent artery occlusion with or without bypass surgery [6,7]. In 2021, we reported our experience on the use of flow diversion stents for large or giant aneurysms [5], demonstrating a relatively low complete occlusion rate (57.1%) and a high complication rate (17.1%) compared to other studies [8–12]. Since then, we have treated a larger patient population and extended the follow-up period, resulting in a significant accumulation of data. This study aims to present updated results and analyze the factors contributing to treatment outcomes after flow diversion. Additionally, with increased experience, we have observed improvements in treatment outcomes, including better aneurysm occlusion rates and reduced complications. By sharing our decade-long experience, we aim to contribute to the optimization of flow diversion stent protocols and improve treatment efficacy.

2. Methods

This study received approval from the institutional review board (IRB File No. 2021-01-176-001) of our institution. We conducted a review of the medical records of patients who underwent flow diversion for intracranial aneurysms at our facility from July 2014 to August 2023. The decision for flow diversion treatment was made based on multidisciplinary team discussions involving neurosurgeons and interventional neuroradiologists, as well as patient preferences. The study population included individuals with unruptured aneurysms in both the anterior and posterior circulation. Patients who were lost to follow-up and had less than 12 months of angiographic follow-up before achieving complete aneurysm occlusion without adverse events were excluded from the analysis, whereas patients who experienced any type of safety outcome were included in the analysis despite having less than 12 months of angiographic follow-up. Clinical data such as age, sex, medical history, and results of platelet reactivity testing were obtained from the medical records of the patients included in the study. The diameter and neck size of the aneurysms were assessed using three-dimensional digital subtraction angiography (DSA), with the maximum value of each dimension recorded. For aneurysms containing luminal thrombi, the diameter was measured as the outer-to-outer diameter on pre-treatment magnetic resonance imaging (MRI).

2.1. Interventions and Follow-Up

All patients received premedication with a dual antiplatelet regimen consisting of either 100 mg aspirin and 75 mg clopidogrel for 5 to 14 days or a loading dose of 300 mg aspirin and clopidogrel for 1 to 2 days prior to the flow diversion procedure. Platelet reactivity was assessed using the VerifyNow Assay (Accumetrics Inc., San Diego, CA, USA). For patients exhibiting clopidogrel hyporesponsiveness (P2Y12 reaction units > 230), ticlopidine (250 mg) was administered twice daily as an alternative. The dual antiplatelet therapy continued for 6 months post-procedure, followed by a single antiplatelet agent for an additional 6 months.

Three types of commercial flow diversion systems were used: the Pipeline Embolization Device (Flex and Flex with Shield technology, Medtronic, Irvine, CA, USA), the Derivo Embolization Device (Acandis GmbH & Co, KG, Pforzheim, Germany), and the Surpass Flow Diverter (Streamline and Evolve, Stryker Neurovascular, CA, USA). The choice of device was based on the operator's preference. Post-procedural MRI was performed within 5 days of the procedure. Clinical and radiological follow-ups included MRI and/or CT angiography at 6, 12, 18, and 24 months after the procedure and annually thereafter. Follow-up assessments were conducted at the discretion of the attending physician.

2.2. Outcome Measures

Complete aneurysm occlusion was defined as the angiographic occlusion of the target aneurysm at the end of follow-up without significant (>50%) parent artery stenosis, major adverse events, or the need for additional treatment. Safety outcomes included hemorrhagic stroke, major ischemic stroke (defined as an increase of $\geq$4 points on the National Institutes of Health Stroke Scale), partial or complete stent thrombosis, and all-cause mortality. Significant enlargement of the target aneurysm and unfavorable functional outcomes were also assessed. As previously described in our study, significant enlargement of the target aneurysm was defined as a follow-up aneurysm volume exceeding 125% of the initial aneurysm volume [7]. The aneurysmal diameter was measured on MRI using the outer-to-outer diameter. Functional outcomes were assessed at an outpatient clinic, with unfavorable functional outcomes defined as a modified Rankin Scale score of 3–6 at the last clinical follow-up. Additionally, we compared the baseline characteristics, treatment details, and treatment outcomes between the early group and the recent group, categorized based on the time of the previous study publication.

2.3. Statistical Analyses

Statistical analyses were performed using SPSS Statistics version 25.0 (IBM Corporation, Armonk, NY, USA) and R version 3.4.2 (R Foundation for Statistical Computing, Vienna, Austria). A p value of <0.05 was considered indicative of statistical significance, with all p values based on two-sided tests. Differences in categorical variables between groups were analyzed using the chi-square test with continuity correction, while continuous variables were compared using the T-test. To determine associations between clinical variables and complete aneurysm occlusion, univariate binary logistic regression analysis was conducted. A multivariate logistic regression model, with a significance level set at 0.20, was then used to identify independent predictors. Odds ratios (ORs) and 95% confidence intervals (CIs) were calculated for the identified risk variables. A Cox proportional hazard analysis was performed to assess time-dependent factors influencing complete aneurysm occlusion after flow diversion, also with a significance level set at 0.20. Hazards ratios (HRs) and 95% confidence intervals (CIs) were calculated for the identified risk variables.

3. Results

During the study period, 128 patients with 134 intracranial aneurysms underwent flow diversion treatment. However, 13 patients with 13 intracranial aneurysms were excluded for the following reasons: incomplete angiographic follow-up (n = 11) or intracranial artery dissection without aneurysm formation (n = 2). Consequently, the final analysis included 115 patients with 121 aneurysms.

Table 1 summarizes the clinicoradiological findings of 121 aneurysms; the patients had a mean age of 59.4 ± 12.9 years and 82 (67.8%) were female. Regarding previous treatments, the majority had no prior interventions (113 patients, 93.4%), while two patients (1.7%) had undergone clipping. Additionally, one patient each had distal occlusion and bypass (0.8%) and multiple stents (0.8%). Coil embolization had been performed in four patients (3.3%). The majority of aneurysms were located in the anterior circulation (85 patients, 70.2%). The mean aneurysm diameter was 15.2 ± 7.0 mm, with sizes categorized as <10 mm in 24 patients (19.8%), 10–25 mm in 82 patients (67.8%), and ≥25 mm in 15 patients (12.4%). The mean neck diameter was 8.9 ± 4.8 mm, and 33 patients (27.3%) had an incorporated branch preventing aneurysm isolation after flow diversion.

Table 1. Clinicoradiological findings of the total 121 aneurysms.

Age (year)	59.4 ± 12.9
Female	82 (67.8%)
Previous treatment	
-No	113 (93.4%)
-Clipping	2 (1.7%)
-Distal occlusion, Bypass	1 (0.8%)
-Multiple stents	1 (0.8%)
-Coil embolization	4 (3.3%)
Anterior circulation	85 (70.2%)
Location	
-ICA	75 (62.0%)
-ACA	4 (3.3%)
-MCA	6 (5.0%)

Table 1. *Cont.*

-PCA	1 (0.8%)
-BA	6 (5.0%)
-VA	29 (24.0%)
Non-saccular type	76 (62.8%)
Aneurysm diameter (mm)	15.2 ± 7.0
-<10	24 (19.8%)
-10–25	82 (67.8%)
-≥25	15 (12.4%)
Neck diameter (mm)	8.9 ± 4.8
Incorporated branch	33 (27.3%)
Pre-treatment mRS	
-0	112 (92.6%)
-1	8 (6.6%)
-2	1 (0.8%)
Pre-treatment DAPT	
-On DAPT	4 (3.3%)
-Loading dose	8 (6.6%)
-Scheduled	109 (90.1%)
Pre-treatment DAPT regimen	
-Aspirin + Cilostazol	1 (0.8%)
-Aspirin + Clopidogrel	120 (99.2%)
ARU	445.4 ± 67.7
PRU	177.4 ± 69.5
Post-treatment DAPT	
-Aspirin + Cilostazol	1 (0.8%)
-Aspirin + Clopidogrel	99 (81.8%)
-Aspirin + Ticlopidine	21 (17.4%)
Device	
-Surpass Flow Diverter, Evolve	67 (55.4%)
-Surpass Flow Diverter, Streamline	31 (25.6%)
-Pipeline Embolization Device, Flex	22 (18.2%)
-Derivo Embolization Device	1 (0.8%)
Additional coil	3 (2.5%)
Number of fow diverters used	
-1	116 (95.9%)
-2	5 (4.1%)
Balloon angioplasty	40 (33.1%)
Procedure time (min)	91.1 ± 44.9
Angiographic follow-up (month)	26.0 ± 19.0
Clinical follow-up (month)	29.5 ± 22.2

ICA, internal carotid artery; ACA, anterior cerebral artery; MCA, middle cerebral artery; PCA, posterior cerebral artery; BA, basilar artery; VA, vertebral artery; mRS, modified Rankin Scale score; DAPT, dual antiplatelet therapy; ARU, aspirin resistance unit; PRU, plavix resistance unit.

The devices used were the Surpass Evolve in 67 patients (55.4%), Surpass Streamline in 31 patients (25.6%), Pipeline Embolization Device in 22 patients (18.2%), and Derivo Embolization Device in 1 patient (0.8%), with additional coils used in 3 patients (2.5%). The number of flow diverters used was 1 in 116 patients (95.9%) and 2 in 5 patients (4.1%). Balloon angioplasty was performed in 40 patients (33.1%), and the mean procedure time was 91.1 ± 44.9 min. The mean angiographic follow-up was 26.0 ± 19.0 months, and the mean clinical follow-up was 29.5 ± 22.2 months.

Complete aneurysm occlusion was achieved in 88 patients (72.7%). The mean duration from flow diversion to aneurysm occlusion was 14.7 ± 15.6 months. Safety outcomes were noted in 11 patients (9.1%), including hemorrhagic events in 4 patients (3.3%) with 2 cases of delayed RIPH (1.7%) and 2 cases of delayed rupture with subarachnoid hemorrhage (SAH) (1.6%). Major infarction occurred in four patients (3.3%), with downstream embolic infarction in one patient (0.8%) and covered perforator territory infarction in one patient (0.8%). Stent thrombosis with infarction was observed in two patients (1.7%). Stent thrombosis without infarction was also noted in two patients (1.7%). There was one case of sudden death from an unknown cause (0.8%). Unfavorable functional outcomes were reported in five patients (4.1%); aneurysm enlargement was seen in 14 patients (11.6%). The treatment outcomes are summarized in Table 2.

Table 2. Clinical outcomes of the study subjects.

Complete aneurysm occlusion *	88 (72.7%)
Safety outcomes	11 (9.1%)
Hemorrhagic stroke	4 (3.3%)
Delayed RIPH	2 (1.7%)
Delayed rupture, SAH	2 (1.6%)
Major ischemic stroke †	4 (3.3%)
Downstream embolic infarction	1 (0.8%)
Covered perforator territory infarction	1 (0.8%)
Stent thrombosis	2 (1.7%)
Stent thrombosis without infarction	2 (1.7%)
Sudden death, unknown cause	1 (0.8%)
Aneurysm enlargement ‡	14 (11.6%)
Unfavorable functional outcome §	5 (4.1%)

RIPH, remote intraparenchymal hemorrhage; SAH subarachnoid hemorrhage; * Complete aneurysm occlusion was defined as the angiographic occlusion of the target aneurysm at the end of follow-up, without significant (>50%) parent artery stenosis, major adverse events, or the need for additional treatment; † Major ischemic stroke was defined as an increase of ≥4 points in the National Institutes of Health Stroke Scale score; ‡ Aneurysm enlargement was defined as a follow-up aneurysm volume exceeding 125% of the initial aneurysm volume; § Unfavorable functional outcomes defined as a modified Rankin Scale score of 3–6 at the last clinical follow-up.

Table 3 presents the results of the logistic regression analysis for complete aneurysm occlusion, safety outcomes, and all stroke (hemorrhagic and major ischemic stroke). In the univariate analysis for aneurysm occlusion, significant factors included non-saccular type ($p = 0.048$, OR = 0.49, 95% CI 0.19–0.99), aneurysm diameter ($p < 0.001$, OR = 0.89, 95% CI 0.83–0.95), neck diameter ($p = 0.004$, OR = 0.85, 95% CI 0.77–0.94), and incorporated branch ($p = 0.002$, OR = 0.25, 95% CI 0.11–0.60). Multivariate analysis showed aneurysm diameter ($p = 0.009$, OR = 0.89, 95% CI 0.82–0.97) and incorporated branch ($p = 0.003$, OR = 0.22, 95% CI 0.08–0.59) remained significant. For safety outcomes, univariate analysis identified aneurysm diameter ($p < 0.001$, OR = 1.20, 95% CI 1.09–1.34) as a significant factor. Multivariate analysis confirmed aneurysm diameter ($p = 0.001$, OR = 1.21, 95% CI 1.09–1.37) as significant. For hemorrhagic and major ischemic stroke, univariate analysis indicated aneurysm diameter ($p = 0.003$, OR = 1.18, 95% CI 1.06–1.33) as significant. Multivariate analysis validated aneurysm diameter (p = 0.003, OR = 1.18, 95% CI 1.06–1.33) as a significant factor. Aneurysm diameter is the most important factor, significantly influencing all treatment outcomes, including complete aneurysm occlusion, safety outcomes, and hemorrhagic and ischemic strokes. Figure 1 shows the percentage of each treatment outcome based on the aneurysm diameter, highlighting that larger aneurysms have lower complete aneurysm occlusion rates and higher complication rates.

Table 3. Logistic regression analysis for complete aneurysm occlusion after flow diversion.

	Complete Aneurysm Occlusion *					
	Univariate Analysis			**Multivariate Analysis**		
	***p* Value**	**OR**	**95% CI**	***p* Value**	**OR**	**95% CI**
Age	0.311	0.98	0.95–1.01			
Male	0.552	0.77	0.34–1.83			
Posterior circulation	0.158	0.54	0.23–1.28	0.584	0.71	0.21–2.51
Non-saccular type	0.048	0.44	0.19–0.99	0.663	1.32	0.39–4.74
Aneurysm diameter	<0.001	0.89	0.83–0.95	0.009	0.89	0.82–0.97
Neck diameter	0.001	0.85	0.77–0.94	0.415	0.94	0.81–1.08
Incorporated branch	0.002	0.25	0.11–0.60	0.003	0.22	0.08–0.59
Number of flow diverters used	0.52	0.55	0.09–4.30			
	Safety Outcomes †					
	Univariate analysis			Multivariate analysis		
	p value	OR	95% CI	*p* value	OR	95% CI
Age	0.555	1.02	0.97–1.07			
Male	0.759	1.22	0.30–4.33			
Posterior circulation	0.850	0.88	0.18–3.24			
Non-saccular type	0.220	2.18	0.62–8.02			
Aneurysm diameter	<0.001	1.20	1.09–1.34	0.001	1.21	1.09–1.37
Neck diameter	0.068	1.10	0.99–1.23	0.702	0.98	0.85–1.11
Incorporated branch	0.483	0.57	0.08–2.35			
Number of flow diverters used	0.403	2.65	0.13–20.22			
	Hemorrhagic and Major Ischemic Stroke					
	Univariate analysis			Multivariate analysis		
	p value	OR	95% CI	*p* value	OR	95% CI
Age	0.812	1.01	0.95–1.07			
Male	0.652	0.68	0.10–3.14			
Posterior circulation	0.293	0.32	0.02–1.89			
Non-saccular type	0.443	1.76	0.40–7.79			
Aneurysm diameter	0.003	1.18	1.06–1.33	0.003	1.18	1.06–1.33
Neck diameter	0.477	1.05	0.90–1.18			
Incorporated branch	0.881	0.88	0.12–4.07			
Number of flow diverters used	0.251	3.89	0.19–31.23			

OR, odds ratio; CI, confidence interval; * Complete aneurysm occlusion was defined as the angiographic occlusion of the target aneurysm at the end of follow-up, without significant (>50%) parent artery stenosis, major adverse events, or the need for additional treatment; † Safety outcomes included hemorrhagic stroke, major ischemic stroke (defined as an increase of ≥4 points on the National Institutes of Health Stroke Scale), partial or complete stent thrombosis, and all-cause mortality.

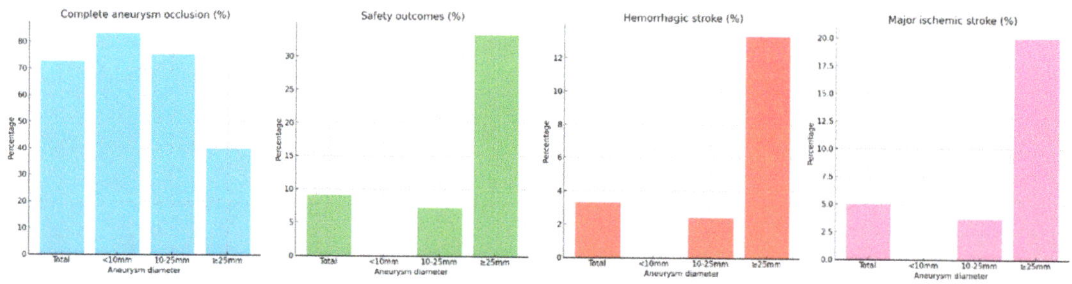

Figure 1. Outcomes of flow diversion treatment stratified by aneurysm diameter.

The results of the Cox proportional hazard analysis are summarized in Table 4 and Figure 2. Univariate analysis identified aneurysm diameter ($p = 0.037$, HR = 0.97, 95% CI 0.94–1.00), neck diameter ($p = 0.006$, HR = 0.93, 95% CI 0.88–0.98), and incorporated branch ($p = 0.001$, HR = 0.39, 95% CI 0.23–0.66) as significant factors. Multivariate analysis confirmed that neck diameter ($p = 0.009$, HR = 0.92, 95% CI 0.87–0.98) and incorporated branch ($p = 0.001$, HR = 0.40, 95% CI 0.24–0.69) remained significant predictors for aneurysm occlusion.

Table 4. Cox proportional hazard analysis for complete aneurysm occlusion after flow diversion.

	Univariate Analysis			Multivariate Analysis		
	p Value	HR	95% CI	*p* Value	HR	95% CI
Age	0.720	1.00	0.98–1.01			
Male	0.375	0.81	0.52–1.28			
Posterior circulation	0.673	0.90	0.56–1.45			
Non-saccular type	0.177	0.73	0.47–1.15			
Aneurysm diameter	0.037	0.97	0.94–1.00			
Neck diameter	0.006	0.93	0.88–0.98	0.009	0.92	0.87–0.98
Incorporated branch	0.001	0.39	0.23–0.66	0.001	0.40	0.24–0.69
Multiple flow diverters use	0.686	0.79	0.25–2.25			

HR, hazards ratio; CI, confidence interval.

Table 5 presents a comparison of baseline characteristics, treatment details, and clinical outcomes between the early group ($n = 47$) and the recent group ($n = 74$). The recent group had a significantly higher proportion of female patients (79.7% vs. 48.9%, $p = 0.001$). Non-saccular aneurysms were more prevalent in the early group (53.2% vs. 27.0%, $p = 0.007$). The early group also had larger mean aneurysm diameters (19.3 $\pm$ 6.2 mm vs. 12.6 $\pm$ 6.3 mm, $p < 0.001$) and neck diameters (10.3 $\pm$ 5.3 mm vs. 7.9 $\pm$ 4.1 mm, $p = 0.005$). Balloon angioplasty was performed more often in the early group (46.8% vs. 24.3%, $p = 0.018$), and their procedures took longer on average (113.4 $\pm$ 52.8 min vs. 77.0 $\pm$ 32.2 min, $p < 0.001$). The recent group had a higher rate of aneurysm occlusion (79.7% vs. 61.7%, $p = 0.050$) and a lower incidence of aneurysm enlargement (2.7% vs. 25.5%, $p < 0.001$). Additionally, the early group experienced higher rates of all strokes (14.9% vs. 1.4%, $p = 0.011$) and hemorrhagic stroke (8.5% vs. 0%, $p = 0.042$).

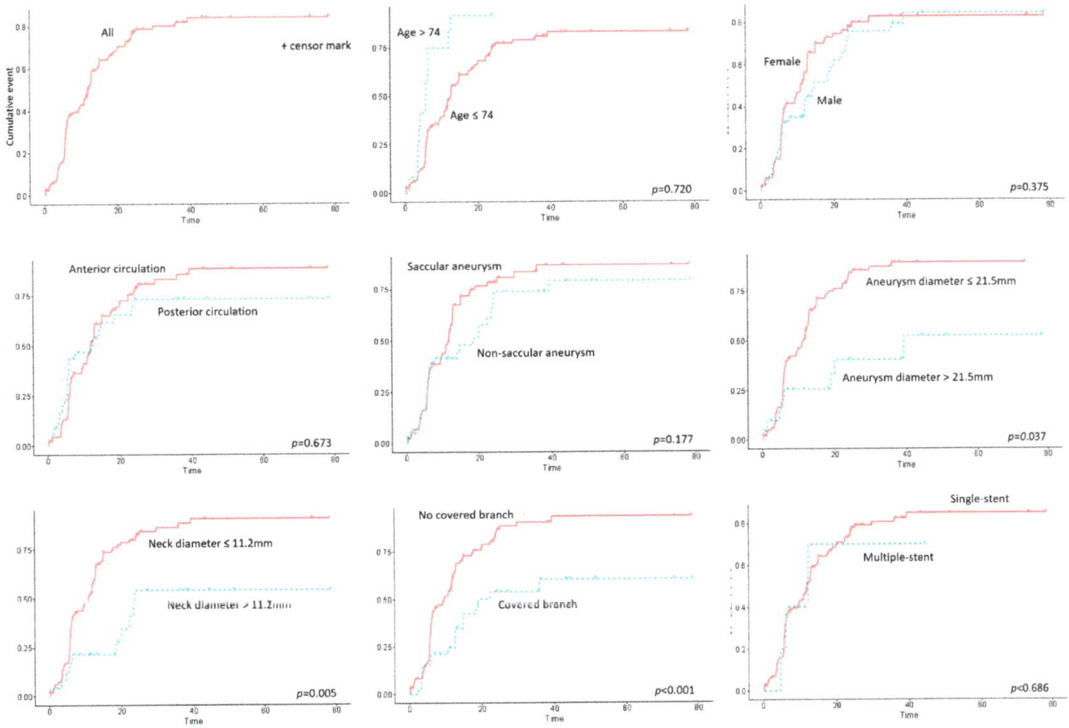

Figure 2. Cumulative event analysis for aneurysm occlusion stratified by various clinical and anatomical factors.

Table 5. Comparison of baseline characteristics, treatment details, and treatment outcomes between early and recent groups.

	Total	Early Group	Recent Group	p Value
	(n = 121)	(n = 47)	(n = 74)	
Age (year)	59.1 ± 13.0	58.7 ± 14.2	59.3 ± 12.2	0.803
Female	82 (67.8%)	23 (48.9%)	59 (79.7%)	0.001
Anterior circulation	85 (70.2%)	29 (61.7%)	56 (75.7%)	0.151
Location				0.058
-ICA	75 (62.0%)	22 (46.8%)	53 (71.6%)	
-ACA	4 (3.3%)	3 (6.4%)	1 (1.4%)	
-MCA	6 (5.0%)	4 (8.5%)	2 (2.7%)	
-PCA	1 (0.8%)	1 (2.1%)	0 (0.0%)	
-BA	6 (5.0%)	2 (4.3%)	4 (5.4%)	
-VA	29 (24.0%)	15 (31.9%)	14 (18.9%)	
Non-saccular type	45 (37.2%)	25 (53.2%)	20 (27.0%)	0.007

Table 5. *Cont.*

	Total	Early Group	Recent Group	*p* Value
Aneurysm diameter (mm)	15.2 ± 7.0	19.3 ± 6.2	12.6 ± 6.3	<0.001
Neck diameter (mm)	8.9 ± 4.8	10.3 ± 5.3	7.9 ± 4.1	0.005
Incorporated branch	33 (27.3%)	17 (36.2%)	16 (21.6%)	0.123
Device				<0.001
-Surpass Flow Diverter, Streamline	31 (25.6%)	31 (66.0%)	0 (0.0%)	
-Pipeline Embolization Device, Flex	22 (18.2%)	13 (27.7%)	9 (12.2%)	
-Surpass Flow Diverter, Evolve	67 (55.4%)	3 (6.4%)	64 (86.5%)	
-Derivo Embolization Device	1 (0.8%)	0 (0.0%)	1 (1.4%)	
Balloon angioplasty	40 (33.1%)	22 (46.8%)	18 (24.3%)	0.018
Procedure time (min)	91.1 ± 44.9	113.4 ± 52.8	77.0 ± 32.2	<0.001
Complete aneurysm occlusion *	88 (72.7%)	29 (61.7%)	59 (79.7%)	0.050
Aneurysm enlargement †	14 (11.6%)	12 (25.5%)	2 (2.7%)	<0.001
Safety outcomes ‡	11 (9.1%)	8 (17.0%)	3 (4.1%)	0.036
All stroke	8 (6.6%)	7 (14.9%)	1 (1.4%)	0.011
-Hemorrhagic stroke	4 (3.3%)	4 (8.5%)	0 (0.0%)	0.042
-Major ischemic stroke §	4 (3.3%)	3 (6.4%)	1 (1.4%)	0.324

ICA, internal carotid artery; ACA, anterior cerebral artery; MCA, middle cerebral artery; PCA, posterior cerebral artery; BA, basilar artery; VA, vertebral artery; * Complete aneurysm occlusion was defined as the angiographic occlusion of the target aneurysm at the end of follow-up, without significant (>50%) parent artery stenosis, major adverse events, or the need for additional treatment; † Aneurysm enlargement was defined as a follow-up aneurysm volume exceeding 125% of the initial aneurysm volume; ‡ Safety outcomes included hemorrhagic stroke, major ischemic stroke (defined as an increase of ≥4 points on the National Institutes of Health Stroke Scale), partial or complete stent thrombosis, and all-cause mortality; § Major ischemic stroke was defined as an increase of ≥4 points in the National Institutes of Health Stroke Scale score.

4. Discussion

Our study provides a detailed analysis of flow diversion treatment outcomes for intracranial aneurysms, focusing on factors affecting complete aneurysm occlusion and safety outcomes. The complete aneurysm occlusion rate of 72.7% was consistent with that observed in previous large cohort studies [8–13]. The safety outcomes, with a complication rate of 9.1%, reflect the inherent risks associated with the procedure but also highlight areas for potential improvement in patient management and pre-procedural planning. Notably, the recent group exhibited a lower complication rate of 4.1%, suggesting that careful case selection and appropriate procedural techniques can significantly enhance patient safety. In a meta-analysis encompassing 29 studies and 1654 aneurysms, Brinjikji et al. reported that subarachnoid hemorrhage from a delayed aneurysm rupture and ischemic stroke occurred in 4% and 6% of patients, respectively, following flow diversion treatment [3]. These complications were notably more frequent in patients with large and giant aneurysms. Another recent meta-analysis indicates that unruptured non-saccular aneurysms in the posterior or distal anterior circulation can be effectively treated with flow diversion, despite notable complication rates (15% ischemic events, 8% morbidity). Larger aneurysms (>10 mm) are associated with higher risks of adverse events [4]. In our study, the mean aneurysm diameter was 15.2 ± 7.0 mm, with 62.8% being non-saccular aneurysms and 38% located in the posterior or distal anterior circulation. Given this composition, our study results are favorable and reaffirm the efficacy of flow diversion for these complex aneurysms.

Technological advancements in flow diversion devices and increased experience in high-volume centers have shown that treatment outcomes are significantly influenced by case selection rather than the stent deployment technique itself [14,15]. From this standpoint, case selection is the most critical factor for treatment outcomes and understanding predictors of favorable outcomes is crucial. Previous studies have identified several predictors, consistently highlighting aneurysm size, the presence of an incorporated vessel, and the location of the aneurysm, particularly if it is distal or posterior [3–5,16–18]. In the present study, logistic regression analysis revealed significant predictors for aneurysm occlusion, including aneurysm diameter and the presence of an incorporated vessel. Aneurysm diameter was also a significant predictor for safety outcomes and stroke events. The Cox proportional hazard analysis provided additional insights into the time-dependent factors influencing aneurysm occlusion. Neck diameter and the presence of an incorporated branch were significant predictors. These results further emphasize the importance of aneurysm morphology in determining treatment success.

4.1. Comparison between Early and Recent Treatment Groups

Our comparison between the early and recent treatment groups revealed significant improvements in outcomes over time, driven by several key factors. As our experience with flow diversion procedures grew, so did our technical proficiency. This is clearly demonstrated by the decreased procedure time in the recent group, averaging 77.0 min compared to 113.4 min in the early group. This reduction in procedure time underscores the increased efficiency and skill development we achieved with continued practice and familiarity with the technique. Another major contributor to the improved outcomes is the advancement in flow diverter devices. The newer devices we adopted over time offer enhanced deliverability and safety features that have significantly bolstered the effectiveness of the treatment. These technological advancements have allowed us to perform the procedures with greater precision and reliability, thereby improving patient outcomes [14,19]. However, the most significant factor contributing to the better results in the recent group is our refined patient selection process. Initially, our selection criteria were broader and our understanding of the factors leading to unfavorable outcomes was less developed. Over time, insights gained from our earlier studies, which identified critical factors such as aneurysm diameter, incorporated branches, and parent vessel angle, allowed us to hone our criteria. This refinement has enabled us to select patients who are more likely to benefit from flow diversion, thereby enhancing overall outcomes and minimizing complications.

4.2. Implications for Clinical Practice

The identification of significant predictors for both treatment success and safety outcomes can inform patient selection criteria, helping clinicians identify those who are most likely to benefit from flow diversion. Flow diversion is a highly valuable treatment option for cerebral aneurysms; however, it is not universally applicable to all complex aneurysm cases. When flow diversion fails, particularly in cases of aneurysm enlargement, delayed rupture, or clinical deterioration, the subsequent treatment options are limited. These often include additional flow diverter deployment or parent artery occlusion with or without bypass surgery. Therefore, it is crucial to consider alternative conventional treatments when unfavorable outcomes are anticipated with flow diversion [20]. However, despite careful consideration and meticulous inspection, finding a promising treatment option for complex aneurysms is difficult and sometimes even impossible. According to the results of our analysis, large or giant aneurysms with wide necks and incorporated branches present significant concerns regarding safety outcomes and treatment efficacy after flow diversion. Although the non-saccular type did not demonstrate statistical significance in the present study, it could be a potential factor associated with unfavorable outcomes. This type may enhance the impact of other poor outcome factors, such as large size and incorporated branches, particularly when they coexist. However, the present study had limitations in fully elucidating this relationship. When technically feasible, our center has increasingly opted for surgical treatment options for such aneurysms compared to the early stage of flow diversion. Since most of these aneurysms are unclippable, surgical options often involve parent artery trapping with bypass or hybrid techniques. We plan to address this topic in a future report.

4.3. Limitations

This study has several limitations. Conducted at a single center, its findings may not be generalizable to other settings. The retrospective design introduces potential biases due to incomplete or missing data and limits the ability to establish causality. The follow-up period, although long, might still miss late complications or recurrences.

5. Conclusions

In conclusion, the combination of increased technical proficiency, advancements in flow diverter devices, and refined patient selection criteria has led to significant improvements in the success of flow diversion treatments over time. These enhancements have collectively contributed to better aneurysm occlusion rates and reduced complication rates, demonstrating the value of experience, technological innovation, and strategic patient selection in optimizing treatment outcomes.

Author Contributions: T.K.J.: Data curation, Formal analysis, Visualization, Writing—original draft. J.Y.Y.: Conceptualization, Methodology. K.H.K.: Resources. J.-S.K.: Resources. P.J.: Conceptualization, Resources, Supervision. All authors have read and agreed to the published version of the manuscript.

Funding: This research received no external funding.

Institutional Review Board Statement: The study was approved by the Institutional Review Board (IRB) of Samsung Medical Center. The IRB file number is SMC 2021-01-176-001, and the approval date is 8 February 2021.

Informed Consent Statement: A waiver of consent was approved by the institutional review board (IRB File No. 2021–01-176–001). This study involves no more than minimal risk to the subject and the waiver will.

Data Availability Statement: The data presented in this study are available on request from the corresponding author due to ethical restrictions. The data contain sensitive patient information, and sharing it publicly could compromise patient confidentiality and violate privacy laws. Therefore, we can only provide the data to researchers who submit a reasonable request and agree to comply with the ethical guidelines and privacy regulations applicable to this data.

Conflicts of Interest: The authors declare no competing interests.

References

1. Becske, T.; Kallmes, D.F.; Saatci, I.; McDougall, C.G.; Szikora, I.; Lanzino, G.; Moran, C.J.; Woo, H.H.; Lopes, D.K.; Berez, A.L.; et al. Pipeline for Uncoilable or Failed Aneurysms: Results from a Multicenter Clinical Trial. *Radiology* **2013**, *267*, 858–868. [CrossRef] [PubMed]
2. Chancellor, B.; Raz, E.; Shapiro, M.; Tanweer, O.; Nossek, E.; Riina, H.A.; Nelson, P.K. Flow Diversion for Intracranial Aneurysm Treatment: Trials Involving Flow Diverters and Long-Term Outcomes. *Neurosurgery* **2020**, *86*, S36–S45. [CrossRef] [PubMed]
3. Brinjikji, W.; Murad, M.H.; Lanzino, G.; Cloft, H.J.; Kallmes, D.F. Endovascular treatment of intracranial aneurysms with flow diverters: A meta-analysis. *Stroke* **2013**, *44*, 442–447. [CrossRef] [PubMed]
4. Cagnazzo, F.; Lefevre, P.H.; Derraz, I.; Dargazanli, C.; Gascou, G.; di Carlo, D.T.; Perrini, P.; Ahmed, R.; Hak, J.F.; Riquelme, C.; et al. Flow-Diversion Treatment for Unruptured Nonsaccular Intracranial Aneurysms of the Posterior and Distal Anterior Circulation: A Meta-Analysis. *AJNR Am. J. Neuroradiol.* **2020**, *41*, 134–139. [CrossRef] [PubMed]
5. Jee, T.K.; Yeon, J.Y.; Kim, K.H.; Kim, J.S.; Hong, S.C.; Jeon, P. Treatment Outcomes After Single-Device Flow Diversion for Large or Giant Aneurysms. *World Neurosurg.* **2021**, *153*, e36–e45. [CrossRef] [PubMed]
6. Salem, M.M.; Sweid, A.; Kuhn, A.L.; Dmytriw, A.A.; Gomez-Paz, S.; Maragkos, G.A.; Waqas, M.; Parra-Farinas, C.; Salehani, A.; Adeeb, N.; et al. Repeat Flow Diversion for Cerebral Aneurysms Failing Prior Flow Diversion: Safety and Feasibility From Multicenter Experience. *Stroke* **2022**, *53*, 1178–1189. [CrossRef] [PubMed]
7. Jee, T.K.; Yeon, J.Y.; Kim, K.H.; Kim, J.S.; Jeon, P. Evaluation of the Significance of Persistent Remnant Filling and Enlargement After Flow Diversion for Intracranial Aneurysms. *World Neurosurg.* **2024**, *184*, e144–e153. [CrossRef] [PubMed]
8. Bender, M.T.; Colby, G.P.; Lin, L.M.; Jiang, B.; Westbroek, E.M.; Xu, R.; Campos, J.K.; Huang, J.; Tamargo, R.J.; Coon, A.L. Predictors of cerebral aneurysm persistence and occlusion after flow diversion: A single-institution series of 445 cases with angiographic follow-up. *J. Neurosurg.* **2018**, *130*, 259–267. [CrossRef] [PubMed]

9. Oishi, H.; Teranishi, K.; Yatomi, K.; Fujii, T.; Yamamoto, M.; Arai, H. Flow Diverter Therapy Using a Pipeline Embolization Device for 100 Unruptured Large and Giant Internal Carotid Artery Aneurysms in a Single Center in a Japanese Population. *Neurol. Med.-Chir.* **2018**, *58*, 461–467. [CrossRef] [PubMed]
10. Madaelil, T.P.; Grossberg, J.A.; Howard, B.M.; Cawley, C.M.; Dion, J.; Nogueira, R.G.; Haussen, D.C.; Tong, F.C. Aneurysm Remnants after Flow Diversion: Clinical and Angiographic Outcomes. *AJNR Am. J. Neuroradiol.* **2019**, *40*, 694–698. [CrossRef]
11. Kallmes, D.F.; Brinjikji, W.; Boccardi, E.; Ciceri, E.; Diaz, O.; Tawk, R.; Woo, H.; Jabbour, P.; Albuquerque, F.; Chapot, R.; et al. Aneurysm Study of Pipeline in an Observational Registry (ASPIRe). *Interv. Neurol.* **2016**, *5*, 89–99. [CrossRef]
12. Liu, J.M.; Zhou, Y.; Li, Y.; Li, T.; Leng, B.; Zhang, P.; Liang, G.; Huang, Q.; Yang, P.F.; Shi, H.; et al. Parent Artery Reconstruction for Large or Giant Cerebral Aneurysms Using the Tubridge Flow Diverter: A Multicenter, Randomized, Controlled Clinical Trial (PARAT). *AJNR Am. J. Neuroradiol.* **2018**, *39*, 807–816. [CrossRef]
13. Martinez-Galdamez, M.; Lamin, S.M.; Lagios, K.G.; Liebig, T.; Ciceri, E.F.; Chapot, R.; Stockx, L.; Chavda, S.; Kabbasch, C.; Farago, G.; et al. Treatment of intracranial aneurysms using the pipeline flex embolization device with shield technology: Angiographic and safety outcomes at 1-year follow-up. *J. Neurointerv. Surg.* **2019**, *11*, 396–399. [CrossRef]
14. Jee, T.K.; Yeon, J.Y.; Kim, K.H.; Kim, J.S.; Hong, S.C.; Jeon, P. Early clinical experience of using the Surpass Evolve flow diverter in the treatment of intracranial aneurysms. *Neuroradiology* **2022**, *64*, 343–351. [CrossRef]
15. Bonney, P.A.; Connor, M.; Fujii, T.; Singh, P.; Koch, M.J.; Stapleton, C.J.; Mack, W.J.; Walcott, B.P. Failure of Flow Diverter Therapy: Predictors and Management Strategies. *Neurosurgery* **2020**, *86*, S64–S73. [CrossRef] [PubMed]
16. Bae, H.J.; Park, Y.K.; Cho, D.Y.; Choi, J.H.; Kim, B.S.; Shin, Y.S. Predictors of the Effects of Flow Diversion in Very Large and Giant Aneurysms. *AJNR Am. J. Neuroradiol.* **2021**, *42*, 1099–1103. [CrossRef]
17. Rouchaud, A.; Brinjikji, W.; Lanzino, G.; Cloft, H.J.; Kadirvel, R.; Kallmes, D.F. Delayed hemorrhagic complications after flow diversion for intracranial aneurysms: A literature overview. *Neuroradiology* **2016**, *58*, 171–177. [CrossRef] [PubMed]
18. Daou, B.; Atallah, E.; Chalouhi, N.; Starke, R.M.; Oliver, J.; Montano, M.; Jabbour, P.; Rosenwasser, R.H.; Tjoumakaris, S.I. Aneurysms with persistent filling after failed treatment with the Pipeline embolization device. *J. Neurosurg.* **2018**, *130*, 1376–1382. [CrossRef] [PubMed]
19. Issa, R.; Al-Homedi, Z.; Syed, D.H.; Aziz, W.; Al-Omari, B. Surpass Evolve Flow Diverter for the Treatment of Intracranial Aneurysm: A Systematic Review. *Brain Sci.* **2022**, *12*, 810. [CrossRef] [PubMed]
20. Acerbi, F.; Mazzapicchi, E.; Falco, J.; Vetrano, I.G.; Restelli, F.; Faragò, G.; La Corte, E.; Bonomo, G.; Bersano, A.; Canavero, I.; et al. The Role of Bypass Surgery for the Management of Complex Intracranial Aneurysms in the Anterior Circulation in the Flow-Diverter Era: A Single-Center Series. *Brain Sci.* **2022**, *12*, 1339. [CrossRef] [PubMed]

brain sciences

MDPI

Article

The Use of Technology-Based Simulation among Medical Students as a Global Innovative Solution for Training

Francesco Guerrini [1], Luca Bertolino [2], Adrian Safa [2], Matilde Pittarello [2], Anna Parisi [2], Ludovica Vittoria Beretta [2], Elena Zambelli [2], Francesca Totis [2], Giovanni Campanaro [2], Lorenzo Pavia [2], Giannantonio Spena [1], Federico Nicolosi [3] and Franco Servadei [2,4,*]

1 Unit of Neurosurgery, Department of Head & Neck Surgery, Fondazione Policlinico IRCCS San Matteo, 27100 Pavia, Italy; frague21@gmail.com (F.G.)

2 Department of Biomedical Sciences, Humanitas University, 20090 Milan, Italy; luca.bertolino@st.hunimed.eu (L.B.); elena.zambelli@st.hunimed.eu (E.Z.)

3 Department of Medicine and Surgery, University of Milano-Bicocca, 20900 Milan, Italy

4 Department of Neurosurgery, IRCCS Humanitas Research Hospital, Rozzano, 20089 Milan, Italy

* Correspondence: franco.servadei@hunimed.eu

Abstract: Background: Technological advancements have been rapidly integrated within the neurosurgical education track since it is a high-risk specialty with little margin for error. Indeed, simulation and virtual reality during training can improve surgical performance and technical skills. Our study aims to investigate the impact of neurosurgical technology-based simulation activities on medical students. Methods and Materials: The "Suturing Mission–The Symposium" was a three-day event held at Humanitas University. Participants had access to live-streamed conferences held by worldwide experts in several fields of neurosurgery and practical simulations of dura mater sutures, microvascular anastomosis, and augmented reality neurosurgical approaches. An anonymous survey was conducted at the beginning and end of the event. Results: 141 medical students with a mean age of 21 participated. After the course, 110 participants (77.5%) showed interest in pursuing a surgical path, with a great prevalence in those who had planned to have a surgical career before the event (88.7% vs. 41.4%, $p < 0.001$). Participants were also asked about their comfort levels while handling surgical instruments, and a good outcome was reached in 72.7% of participants, with a significant difference between those who had previously attended a suture course (87.8% vs. 66.3%, $p = 0.012$). Conclusion: Training sessions on surgical simulators were effective in increasing participants' interest in pursuing a surgical path, improving their understanding of postgraduate orientation, and boosting their confidence with surgical instruments.

Keywords: education; neurosurgery; surgical training; technical skills; simulation

1. Introduction

Nowadays, neurosurgery does not represent a surgical specialty only, but also a fascinating and technologically growing field that it is often feared by medical students due to the traditional stereotypes of a technically complex, competitive field, with male preponderance [1], a high workload, risk of burnout [2], and susceptibility to litigation [3].

A possible, but difficult, solution could be increasing exposure to the neurosurgical environment before graduation [4–6]. Moreover, educational activities, interest-based groups, and collaborations are also suggested as a solution to ameliorate the perception and exposure of medical students to neurosurgery [4].

Technological advancements have been rapidly integrated with the neurosurgical field since it is a high-risk specialty with little margin for error. Indeed, it has been demonstrated that simulation and virtual reality during training can not only improve surgical performance and technical skills but also increase confidence in residents.

The integration of simulation could be useful in both the training and the performance of surgical procedures, allowing a faster learning curve, improving conceptual understanding of complex anatomy, and enhancing visuospatial skills for the developing neurosurgeon [5].

An ex vivo simulation study has been proven effective for improving students' motivation to pursue a neurosurgical career [6]. However, there is a lack of published experiences with technology-based new simulation settings to expose medical students to some aspects of neurosurgery and contribute to shaping their perspectives and career choices. Introducing technology-based simulations early in medical school could bridge the gap between theory and practice in neurosurgery. This approach can help students make informed decisions about their career path, potentially reducing residency dropouts.

For this reason, we have conducted a study aiming to investigate the impact of neurosurgical technology-based simulation activity on medical students with no restriction of age or background, with respect to their careers and awareness of personal interests and manual abilities.

2. Materials and Methods

The "Suturing Mission–The Symposium" was a three-day event held at Humanitas University, Pieve Emanuele, Milan, Italy from the 11th to the 13th of November 2022, organized by a nonprofit network called Mission:Brain (https://www.missionbrain.org/about, accessed on 1 February 2023). Original data regarding students' participation and survey results are reported in Supplementary Materials. The funds raised by the tickets required to participate are entirely devoted to sustaining similar events in other countries with limited facilities, where Mission:Brain associations are present. The symposium involves a series of both in-person and virtual conferences, internationally live-streamed, held by worldwide experts in several fields of neurosurgery and practical hands-on sessions of training on cadaver-free simulation technologies, developed and furnished via a free unlimited grant by UpSurgeOn, an Italian company based in Assago, Milan, Italy. Through voluntary recruitment, we have enrolled medical students from various academic years, from 1st-year students to 6th-year students. For the practical sessions, participants were all randomly divided into small groups and had the opportunity to rotate between two different stands where they could perform and practice dura mater sutures and microvascular anastomosis with microsuturing instruments (Figure 1). All the students performed the same task in the same way. In the dura mater suture session, they all had to perform a suture of a rectangular flap using a simple knot for two sides and a continuous knot for the third one, using a 4-0 suture thread (Figure 2). In the vessel anastomosis session, they all performed a side-to-side anastomosis via simple knot using an 8-0 suture thread (Figure 3). Mycro is the name of the simulator employed in this activity. It is a pocket-sized training kit for microsurgical techniques, which consists of a box with a high-fidelity representation of the brain, on which it is possible to integrate a membrane representing the dura mater (Figure 2) or a high-fidelity reproduction of a vessel (Figure 3). At a third station, they also had the opportunity to deepen their knowledge of neuroanatomy and neurosurgical approaches thanks to augmented reality and specific anatomical models developed by UpSurgeOn that integrate this technology. During each one of the practical sessions, both the suturing of the dura mater and the microvessel anastomosis, the participants were always under the guidance of trained staff and neurosurgery residents.

An anonymous survey was conducted at the beginning and the end of the event. It consisted of 28 questions, both open- and closed-ended. Six sections investigated anagraphical and background data, motivations, and medical and general skills held before and after the event. Missing data led to student exclusion from the final analysis (Tables 1 and 2). Demographics and background data regarding the total number of participants, mean age, year of medical school, orientation, left- or right-handed, and vision problems were gathered. Data regarding any previous attendance of surgical intervention and suture courses were collected to assess the medical skills of the participants before the event.

Participants' general skills were assessed through a Likert-scale from 1 to 5 (1 = Strongly Disagree, 2 = Disagree, 3 = Neutral, 4 = Agree, and 5 = Strongly Agree) and concerned free-time activities sphere. After training on the simulators, participants were asked how much they agree with different statements, using the same scale from 1 to 5.

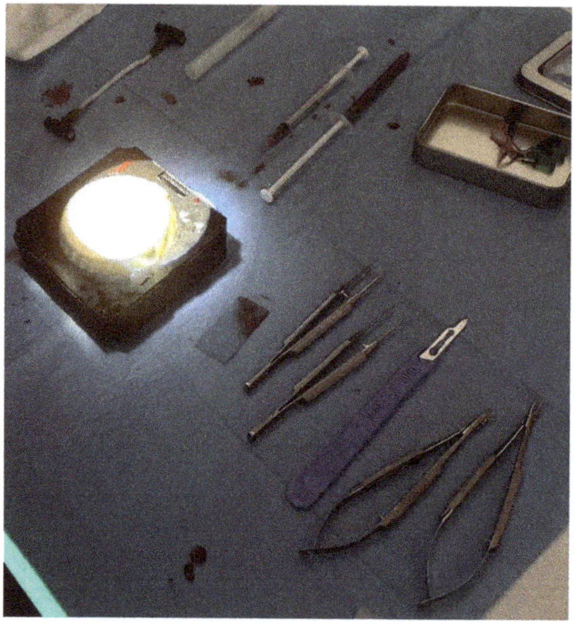

Figure 1. Microsuturing instruments used: micro-scissor, micro-forceps with teeth, micro-forceps without teeth, needle-holder, disposable scalpel, fake blood, and fake blood vessel.

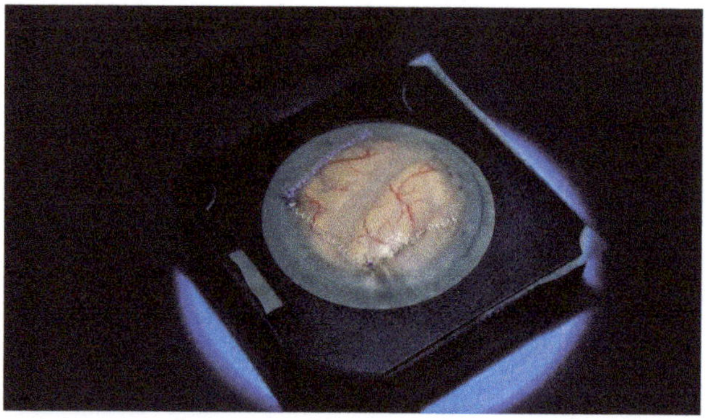

Figure 2. Simulator set for dura mater.

Statistical analyses were performed using R software v4.0.1. Chi-squared test (or Fisher's exact test if applicable) was used to evaluate differences in proportions among subgroups of interest. Values of $p < 0.05$ were considered statistically significant. Data are presented as absolute and relative frequencies if not otherwise specified. A "bad outcome" reflected a score from 1 to 3, while 4 and 5 points were considered a "good outcome".

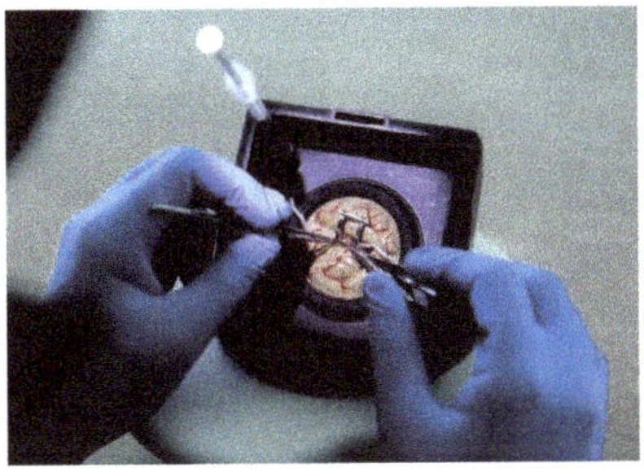

Figure 3. Simulator set for vessel anastomosis.

Table 1. Questions related to personal information and background information.

QUESTION	ANSWERED REQUIRED
PERSONAL INFO	
Age	Open (numerical)
Nationality	Open
STUDIES AND BACKGROUND	
University	Open
Current year of studies	Open (numerical)
High school attended (type)	Open
Interest in pursuing a medical career	Clinical/surgical
If clinical, does it involve neurosciences?	Yes/No
If surgical, which field	Open
Dominant hand	Left/Right
Visual defects	Myopia/Hypermetropia/Astigmatism/None
MOTIVATION	
Why have you chosen to take part in this project?	Multiple choice

Table 2. Questions related to the skills possessed by the participants.

QUESTION	ANSWERED REQUIRED
MEDICAL SKILLS POSSESSED BEFORE THE EVENT	
Seen a surgical operation	Yes/No
Attended a suture technique course	Yes/No
GENERAL SKILLS POSSESED BEFORE THE EVENT	
I know how to play a musical instrument.	Likert scale from 1 to 5
I know how to draw or paint	Likert scale from 1 to 5
I know how to make a sculpture	Likert scale from 1 to 5
I am practical with DIY/gardening	Likert scale from 1 to 5
I am practical with needlework	Likert scale from 1 to 5
I play videogames	Likert scale from 1 to 5
If you play videogames (answer ≥ 3):	
Which kind of videogames?	Open
Have you ever used kinematic sensors?	Yes/No

Table 2. *Cont.*

QUESTION	ANSWERED REQUIRED
POST SIMULATION ASSESMENT	
The event made me realize that I am interested in pursuing a surgical path.	Likert scale from 1 to 5
The event made me realize that I am interested in pursuing a medical path in the neurosciences.	Likert scale from 1 to 5
The event was useful to understand my postgraduate orientation outside of a surgical path.	Likert scale from 1 to 5
The event was useful to understand my postgraduate orientation in the neurosciences' field.	Likert scale from 1 to 5
I would like to join another simulation event.	Likert scale from 1 to 5
I felt comfortable while handling the surgical instruments.	Likert scale from 1 to 5

3. Results

One hundred and forty-one medical students were included in the study. The mean age was 21 years (Table 3). The greater part of them were in their second (39.7%) and third (27.7%) year of medical school program (Table 3).

Table 3. Demographics and specific characteristic of participants.

Number of Participants		141
Mean Age		21
Year of Medical School	1st	10
	2nd	56
	3rd	39
	4th	22
	5th	7
	6th	7
Orientation	Surgical	98
	Clinical	21
	Both	6
Hand	R	127
	L	15
Vision	M	53
	M/A	22
	H	3
	NONE	42
	M/A/H	1
Surgical Intervention	Yes	79
	No	67
Suture Course	Yes	41
	No	105
Kinetic Sensors	Yes	19
	No	49

Before the simulation, specialty preferences were investigated among participants, showing 103 expressing an interest in pursuing a surgical specialty and 29 for a clinical specialty; a common interest in both surgical and clinical residency was present in 6 cases (Table 3) (Figures 4 and 5). Around half of all participants showed a self-inclination for neurosciences, and 54% of them had already assisted in a surgical intervention. (Table 3) (Figures 6 and 7) Myopia and hypermetropia were present in fifty-three and three cases, respectively. Forty-two students had a normal sight. As far as previous training is concerned, 41 students had already attended a suture technique course (Table 3, Figure 6).

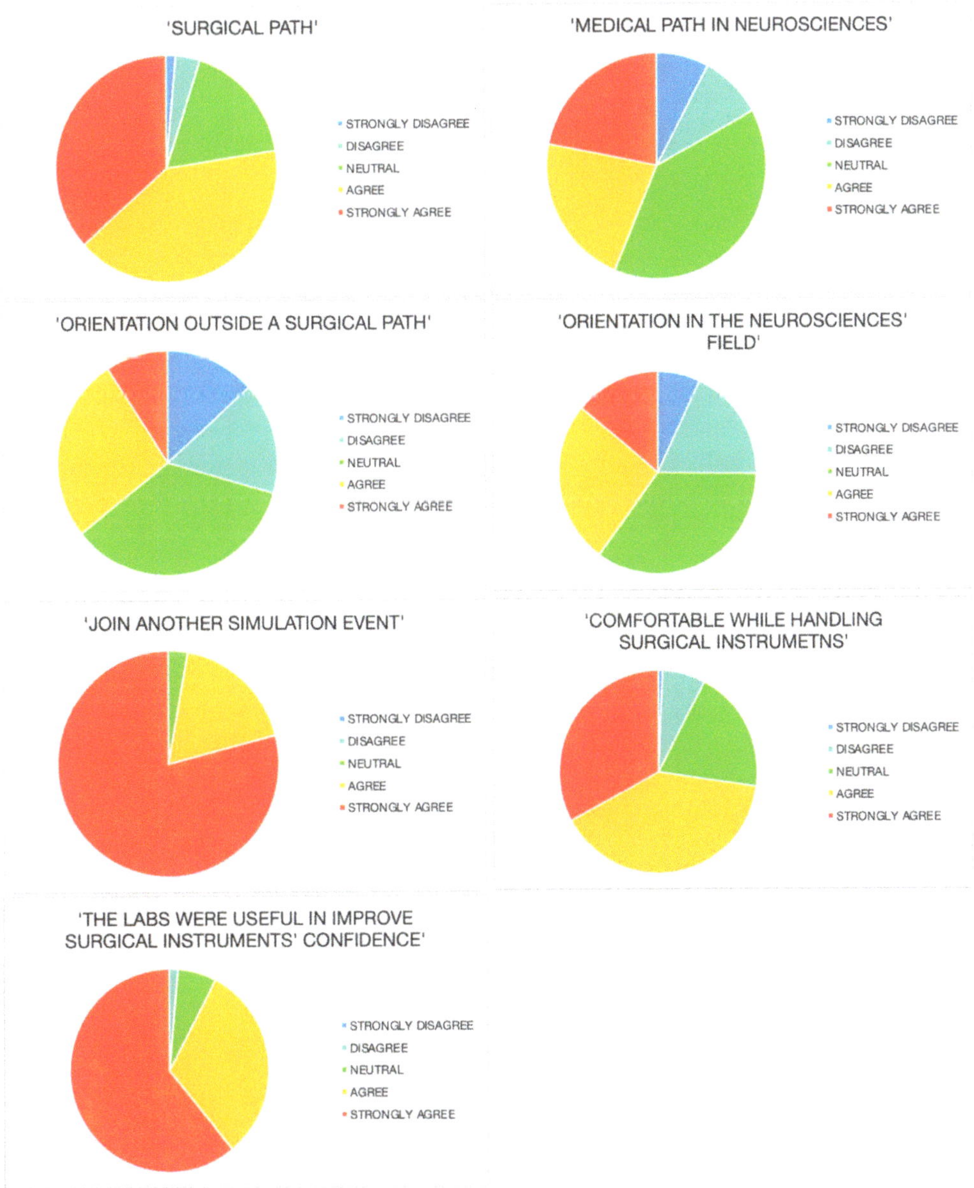

Figure 4. Pie charts representing post-simulation assessment of the participants.

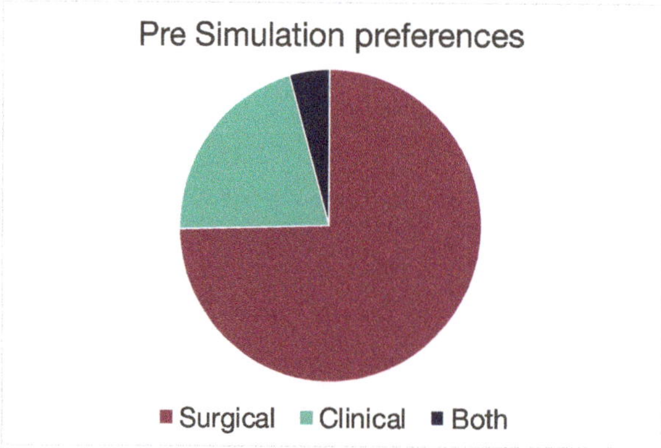

Figure 5. Specialty preference before simulation.

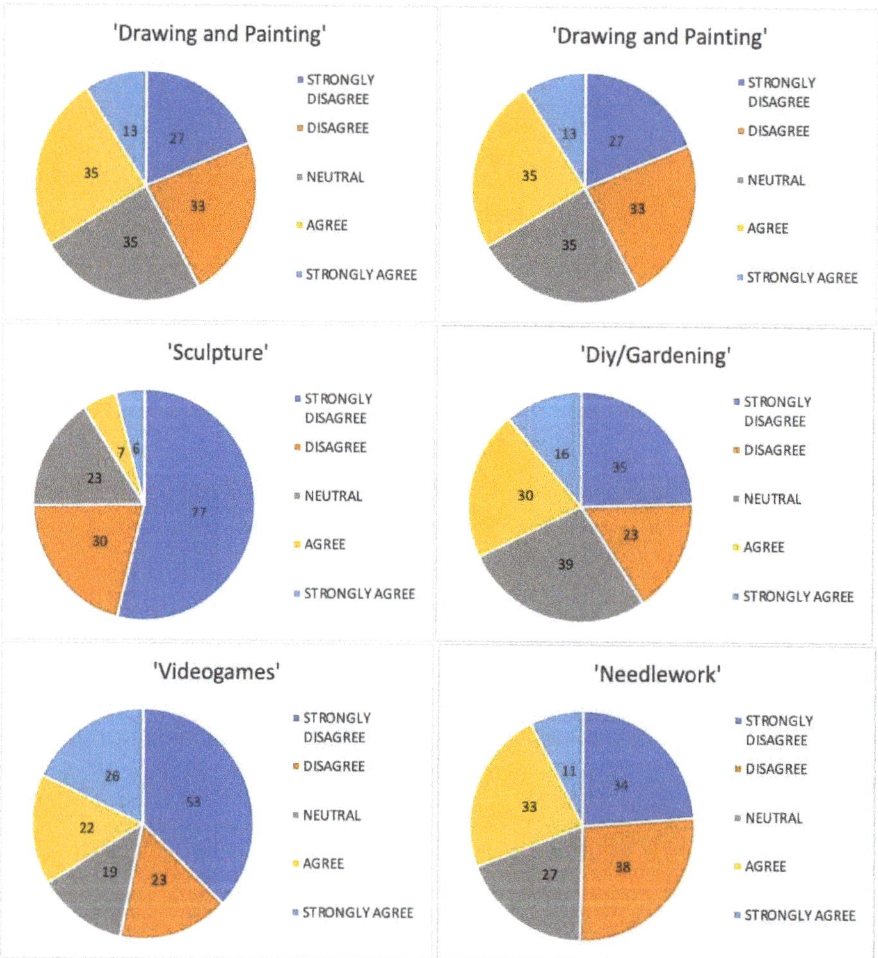

Figure 6. Pie charts representing general skills possessed by the participants before the event.

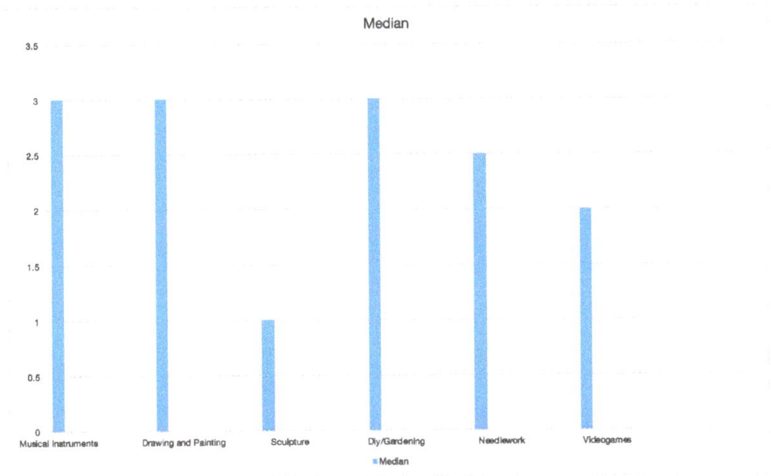

Figure 7. Median value of grades for each general skill assessed.

After the course, 110 participants (77.5%) showed an interest in pursuing a surgical path, with a great prevalence in those who had planned to have a surgical career before the event (87.7% vs. 41.4%, $p < 0.001$) (Table 4, Figure 4).

Table 4. Data regarding the post-simulation assessment organized by pre-course attitude.

The event made me realize that I am interest in pursuing a surgical path			
Precourse Attitude	*Bad outcome (%)*	*Good outcome (%)*	*p value*
Surgical	13 (12.3)	93 (87.8)	***<0.001***
Clinical	17 (58.6)	12 (41.4)	
Both	2 (33.3)	4 (66.6)	
The event made me realize that I am interest in pursuing a medical path in the neurosciences			
Precourse Attitude	*Bad outcome (%)*	*Good outcome (%)*	*p value*
Neuro	26 (32.5)	45 (72.6)	***<0.001***
No neuro	54 (67.5)	17 (27.4)	
The event was useful in understanding my postgraduate orientation outside of a surgical path			
Precourse Attitude	*Bad outcome (%)*	*Good outcome (%)*	*p value*
Surgical	72 (67.9)	34 (32.0)	***0.259***
Clinical	16 (53.3)	14 (46.7)	
Both	3 (50)	3 (50)	
The event was useful in understanding my postgraduate orientation in the neuroscience's field			
Precourse Attitude	*Bad outcome (%)*	*Good outcome (%)*	*p value*
Neuro	34 (47.9)	37 (52.1)	***0.004***
No neuro	52 (72.2)	20 (27.8)	
I would like to join another simulation event			
Precourse Attitude	*Bad outcome (%)*	*Good outcome (%)*	*p value*
Sutures	3 (7.3)	38 (92.6)	***0.072***
No sutures	1 (0.9)	100 (99.0)	

Table 4. *Cont.*

I felt comfortable while handling the surgical instruments			
Precourse Attitude	*Bad outcome (%)*	*Good outcome (%)*	*p value*
Sutures YES	5 (12.2)	36 (87.8)	**0.012**
Sutures NO	34 (33.7)	67 (66.3)	
I felt comfortable while handling the surgical instruments			
Precourse Attitude	*Bad outcome (%)*	*Good outcome (%)*	*p value*
Surgical	26 (24.5)	80 (75.5)	**0.204**
Clinical	12 (40.0)	18 (60.0)	
Both	1 (16.7)	5 (83.3)	

The course reinforced the tendency to follow a medical neurosciences path in students who were interested in this field at the beginning (Table 4). Equally, it strengthened the intention to pursue other fields in the remaining participants (72.6% vs. 27.4%, $p < 0.001$) (Table 4). Moreover, pre-event students' disposition influenced the tendency to follow a general neuroscience pathway (52.1% vs. 27.8%, $p = 0.004$) (Table 4).

When asked if the course was useful in orientating postgraduate pathways outside a surgical field, 92 participants (64.3%) gave a negative answer (Table 5, Figure 4). However, the pre-course specialty orientation of the students did not influence this issue ($p = 0.259$) (Table 4).

Table 5. Data regarding the post-simulation assessment.

The event made me realize that I am interested in pursuing a surgical path			
Grade	*Outcome (%)*	*Grade*	*Outcome (%)*
1	2 (1.4)	Bad	32 (22.5)
2	5 (3.5)		
3	25 (17.6)		
4	58 (40.8)	Good	110 (77.5)
5	52 (36.6)		
The event made me realize that I am interested in pursuing a medical path in neuroscience			
Grade	*Outcome (%)*	*Grade*	*Outcome (%)*
1	11 (7.8)	Bad	80 (56.3)
2	13 (9.2)		
3	56 (39.4)		
4	31 (21.8)	Good	62 (43.7)
5	31 (21.8)		
The event was useful in understanding my postgraduate orientation outside of a surgical path.			
Grade	*Outcome (%)*	*Grade*	*Outcome (%)*
1	19 (13.3)	Bad	92 (64.3)
2	23 (16.1)		
3	50 (35.0)		
4	38 (26.6)	Good	51 (35.7)
5	13 (9.1)		

Table 5. *Cont.*

the event was useful in understanding my postgraduate orientation in the neuroscience's field			
Grade	*Outcome (%)*	*Grade*	*Outcome (%)*
1	10 (7.0)	Bad	86 (60.1)
2	26 (18.2)		
3	50 (35.0)		
4	37 (25.9)	Good	57 (39.9)
5	20 (14.0)		
I would like to join another simulation event			
Grade	*Outcome (%)*	*Grade*	*Outcome (%)*
1	0 (0.0)	Bad	4 (2.8)
2	0 (0.0)		
3	4 (2.8)		
4	26 (18.2)	Good	139 (97.2)
5	113 (79.0)		
I felt comfortable while handling the surgical instruments			
Grade	*Outcome (%)*	*Grade*	*Outcome (%)*
1	1 (0.6)	Bad	39 (27.3)
2	10 (7.0)		
3	28 (19.6)		
4	57 (39.9)	Good	104 (72.7)
5	47 (32.9)		

Participants were also asked about their comfort levels while handling surgical instruments. A good outcome was reached in 72.7% of participants (Table 5, Figure 4), with a significant difference between those who had attended a suturing course previously (87.8% vs. 66.3%, $p = 0.012$) (Table 4).

Finally, 97.2% of students agreed or strongly agreed to attend another simulation course (Table 5, Figure 4).

Participants were also asked about their general skills possessed before the event. Results are reported in Table 6.

Table 6. Data on general skills possessed by the participants before the event.

Musical Instruments			
Grade	*N. of Participants*	*%*	*Median*
1	26	18.2	3
2	25	17.5	
3	22	15.4	
4	41	28.7	
5	29	20.3	

Table 6. *Cont.*

Drawing and Painting			
Grade	*N. of Participants*	%	*Median*
1	27	18.9	3
2	33	23.1	
3	35	24.5	
4	35	24.5	
5	13	9.1	
Sculpture			
Grade	*N. of Participants*	%	*Median*
1	77	53.8	1
2	30	21.0	
3	23	16.1	
4	7	4.9	
5	6	4.2	
Diy/Gardening			
Grade	*N. of Participants*	%	*Median*
1	35	24.5	3
2	23	16.1	
3	39	27.3	
4	30	21.0	
5	16	11.2	
Needlework			
Grade	*N. of Participants*	%	*Median*
1	34	23.8	2.5
2	38	26.6	
3	27	18.9	
4	33	23.1	
5	11	7.7	
Videogames			
Grade	*N. of Participants*	%	*Median*
1	53	37.1	2
2	23	16.1	
3	19	13.3	
4	22	15.4	
5	26	18.2	

4. Discussion

Simulation has always played a central role in human history in order to ameliorate abilities and reduce errors. We have traces dating back to 500 BC reporting simulation games to train decision-making and operational strategies and plan military tactics [7].

Simulation has been employed in many different fields, including aviation, the military, and medicine.

The first successful use of simulation in aviation began in the late 1920s with the Link Trainer, developed by Edwin Link, which allowed pilots to practice their skills in flying "blind" or in instrument training. Standards were implemented in aviation to create reliability in training and evaluation, making it possible to move to the use of predominately simulator-based training methods [8].

It is therefore straightforward to understand how, in a highly demanding, high-risk, technically difficult specialty, such as neurosurgery, the role of simulation plays a crucial role.

Simulation can be aimed at general neurosurgery as well as at specific neurosurgical sub-specialties, such as vascular neurosurgery, minimally invasive neurosurgery, brain tumor resection, pediatric neurosurgery, stereotactic radiosurgery, skull base neurosurgery, spine surgery, and functional neurosurgery [9].

Simulation techniques vary and span from physical models and visual reality, to mixed reality [10] and augmented reality. In the past, physical reality models included both animal and human cadaver models, playing a central role in the training of neurosurgeons but presenting several limitations such as safety risks, ethical regulations in material repairability, and failure to properly represent parameters of alive tissues [11].

Virtual reality models create a virtual world reproduced by recreating sounds and sensory stimuli experienced by the subject, which can be immersive or non-immersive [12]. It can be applied and aimed at multiple purposes in neurosurgery: neuronavigation [13], as a diagnostic tool [14], in neurosurgical training [15], for pain management [16], in rehabilitation [17], and in robotic neurosurgery [18]. The challenges of vital reality in neurosurgery are commonly linked to the technical complexity, applicability, adherence to real-life scenarios, ethics, and costs [19].

Mixed reality models combine a physical and a virtual component, making it possible for the user to interact with digital objects starting from real ones.

Augmented reality represents the physical world, and digital inputs are superimposed on it via a camera [20]. It is less immersive and more accessible than mixed reality, and in neurosurgery, it plays a crucial role in education, surgical planning, and neuronavigation and is growing in importance in spinal surgery [21].

Extend reality simulation tools show wide and heterogeneous applicability in neurosurgery and present a potential tool to seal the gap in neurosurgical training in low-income countries [19].

Given the wide variety of techniques and levels of difficulty provided, simulation systems can be used at various levels of expertise in the training of neurosurgery professionals. Simulation plays a valuable role in the training of residents [22] and in the planning and sub-specialization of neurosurgeons [23].

The role of neurosurgery simulation for medical students has previously been shown to have an educational benefit and impact on student motivation using an ex vivo pig model [6] or reusable microsurgery kits [24].

In this course, we used a peculiar simulation model, in which dura mater and brain reproductions are highly accurate and detailed. We think that a simulator with these attitudes could improve motor acquisition and automate psychomotor skills, in a cheap and risk-free framework [25].

Our study collects opinions from a large cohort of 141 medical students, with no limitations on age, previous experiences, or background. Firstly, the course resulted in being beneficial in helping students orient toward a surgical pathway, above all, in those who had expressed a surgical attitude at the beginning; nevertheless, when they were asked if the event reinforced a postgraduate inclination outside a surgical pathway, 64.3% of participants disagreed with this statement. This data should be read with the fact that 91% of trainees reported increasing confidence in handling surgical instruments, without a difference based on initial orientation. This is a very important finding, as it translates with the fact that such an organized course could, with the help of tutors like trainees or staff neurosurgeons, guide medical students to a postgraduate surgical world. In support of this, there was generalized enthusiasm, with around 80% of participants reporting being interested in taking part in future similar events. Obviously, those who had already attended a suture course felt more comfortable with surgical instruments, as they started at a higher level.

This course was centered on neurosciences, and it emerged from the fact that although only 43.7% of participants agreed or strongly agreed to pursue a postgraduate medical path in neurosciences, a significant difference was found according to pre-course attitudes. In fact, it reinforced the intention of those students who were already interested in this field.

These results are not only encouraging but propose our study as a model to introduce medical students to the surgery and neuroscience worlds. We know that in many medical schools, neurosurgical teaching is limited (12 h altogether in Italy and many other European countries); in some African countries, neurosurgery is completely out of the medical teaching curriculum. Hence, how can we increase the number of neurosurgeons in countries in need if medical students never cross this specialty? [26,27]. The event combined neuroscience conferences and practical simulations, which proved to be an effective way to introduce students to both theoretical and practical aspects of neurosurgery. In fact, early and aware carrier decisions could prove to be beneficial both to students, reinforcing their intention to follow a career in neurological sciences and to bypass stereotypes generally associated with surgery, and to neurosurgery residency programs since an early and more pondered carrier choice could limit the dropout rate from programs. Moreover, this particular training model, due to its low costs, has proven to be a valid training tool for young neurosurgery residents in low–middle-income countries to overcome their limited possibilities [28].

5. Limitations

The main limitations of our study concern the low number of participants and the lack of an objective tool to study the efficacy of the simulator technologies among medical students. Other limitations could be the absence of a control group, due to the setting of our event, and the absence of different staging sessions to better assess the performance of the participants. Moreover, there are potential cofactors, such as individual interests, experiences, educational environment, and background, that may influence the results. In this study we have only evaluated the following: having an interest to pursue a specialty career in a surgical or clinical field before the event, having a pre-event interest in pursuing a clinical career concerning the neurosciences, and whether or not they have participated in a suturing course before the event.

6. Conclusions

Overall, the result of this study shows that the introduction of medical students to the simulation training under the supervision of residents was effective in increasing students' interest in pursuing a surgical and neuroscience path, improving their understanding of postgraduate orientation, and offering an alternative to a significant inclusion in the neurosurgical teaching at medical schools. However, long-term studies should be conducted to evaluate how these outcomes of interest will change and allow the addition of control groups to the simulation-trained cohort.

Supplementary Materials: The following supporting information can be downloaded at: https://www.mdpi.com/article/10.3390/brainsci14070627/s1.

Author Contributions: Conceptualization, F.G., L.B., M.P., A.S., F.T. and G.C.; methodology, L.B., F.G., F.T. and G.C.; formal analysis, F.G.; investigation, F.G. and L.B.; data curation, F.G. and L.B.; writing—original draft preparation, L.B., A.S., M.P., A.P., L.V.B. and E.Z.; writing—review and editing, L.B., M.P., A.S., F.G. and F.S.; visualization, L.B., M.P., A.S. and A.P.; supervision, F.G., F.S., F.N. and G.S.; project administration, L.B., M.P., A.S. and L.P. All authors have read and agreed to the published version of the manuscript.

Funding: This research received no external funding. Neverthess funding were spontaneously collected during the event to allow future similar events to be organized in countries with limited facilities connected to Mission Brain.

Institutional Review Board Statement: Not applicable.

Informed Consent Statement: Not applicable.

Data Availability Statement: The original contributions presented in the study are included in the article/Supplementary Materials; further inquiries can be directed to the corresponding author.

Acknowledgments: The authors thank Marco Viganò for advice and statistical analysis of the survey's data. The authors in particular thank the co-authors Giorgio Ratti, Chiara Punziano, and Anna Dashiell for their contribution in project administration, data curation, and reviewing the article.

Conflicts of Interest: Dr. Nicolosi is the inventor of the technology used in this study, outside the submitted work, and is also the founder and CEO of UpSurgeOn S.r.l. In addition, Dr. Nicolosi has issued a patent for 20705104.6. Dr. Spena is a co-founder of UpSurgeOn S.r.l.

References

1. Hill, C.S.; Dias, L.; Kitchen, N. Perceptions of Neurosurgery: A Survey of Medical Students and Foundation Doctors. *Br. J. Neurosurg.* **2011**, *25*, 261–267. [CrossRef] [PubMed]
2. Tomasello, F. Neurosurgical Recruitment: The Gold Rush. *World Neurosurg.* **2015**, *83*, 37–38. [CrossRef] [PubMed]
3. Nahed, B.V.; Babu, M.A.; Smith, T.R.; Heary, R.F. Malpractice Liability and Defensive Medicine: A National Survey of Neurosurgeons. *PLoS ONE* **2012**, *7*, e39237. [CrossRef] [PubMed]
4. Stumpo, V.; Latour, K.; Traylor, J.I.; Staartjes, V.E.; Giordano, M.; Caccavella, V.M.; Olivi, A.; Ricciardi, L.; Signorelli, F. Medical Student Interest and Recruitment in Neurosurgery. *World Neurosurg.* **2020**, *141*, 448–454.e6. [CrossRef] [PubMed]
5. Bernardo, A. Virtual Reality and Simulation in Neurosurgical Training. *World Neurosurg.* **2017**, *106*, 1015–1029. [CrossRef]
6. Hanrahan, J.; Sideris, M.; Tsitsopoulos, P.P.; Bimpis, A.; Pasha, T.; Whitfield, P.C.; Papalois, A.E. Increasing Motivation and Engagement in Neurosurgery for Medical Students through Practical Simulation-Based Learning. *Ann. Med. Surg.* **2018**, *34*, 75–79. [CrossRef] [PubMed]
7. Smith, R. The Long History of Gaming in Military Training. *Simul. Gaming* **2010**, *41*, 6–19. [CrossRef]
8. Aebersold, M. The History of Simulation and Its Impact on the Future. *AACN Adv. Crit. Care* **2016**, *27*, 56–61. [CrossRef]
9. Rehder, R.; Abd-El-Barr, M.; Hooten, K.; Weinstock, P.; Madsen, J.R.; Cohen, A.R. The Role of Simulation in Neurosurgery. *Childs Nerv. Syst.* **2016**, *32*, 43–54. [CrossRef] [PubMed]
10. Bova, F.J.; Rajon, D.A.; Friedman, W.A.; Murad, G.J.; Hoh, D.J.; Jacob, R.P.; Lampotang, S.; Lizdas, D.E.; Lombard, G.; Lister, J.R. Mixed-Reality Simulation for Neurosurgical Procedures. *Neurosurgery* **2013**, *73*, S138–S145. [CrossRef]
11. Benet, A.; Rincon-Torroella, J.; Lawton, M.T.; González Sánchez, J.J. Novel Embalming Solution for Neurosurgical Simulation in Cadavers: Laboratory Investigation. *J. Neurosurg.* **2014**, *120*, 1229–1237. [CrossRef]
12. Pelargos, P.E.; Nagasawa, D.T.; Lagman, C.; Tenn, S.; Demos, J.V.; Lee, S.J.; Bui, T.T.; Barnette, N.E.; Bhatt, N.S.; Ung, N.; et al. Utilizing Virtual and Augmented Reality for Educational and Clinical Enhancements in Neurosurgery. *J. Clin. Neurosci.* **2017**, *35*, 1–4. [CrossRef] [PubMed]
13. Eric, L.; Grimson, W.; Kikinis, R.; Jolesz, F.A.; Mc, L.; Black, P. Image-Guided Surgery. *Sci. Am.* **1999**, *280*, 62–69. [CrossRef] [PubMed]
14. Mitha, A.P.; Almekhlafi, M.A.; Janjua, M.J.J.; Albuquerque, F.C.; McDougall, C.G. Simulation and Augmented Reality in Endovascular Neurosurgery: Lessons From Aviation. *Neurosurgery* **2013**, *72*, A107–A114. [CrossRef] [PubMed]
15. Kockro, R.A.; Stadie, A.; Schwandt, E.; Reisch, R.; Charalampaki, C.; Ng, I.; Yeo, T.T.; Hwang, P.; Serra, L.; Perneczky, A. A collaborative virtual reality environment for neurosurgical planning and training. *Oper. Neurosurg.* **2007**, *61*, 379–391. [CrossRef] [PubMed]
16. Pourmand, A.; Davis, S.; Marchak, A.; Whiteside, T.; Sikka, N. Virtual Reality as a Clinical Tool for Pain Management. *Curr. Pain Headache Rep.* **2018**, *22*, 53. [CrossRef] [PubMed]
17. Gourlay, D.; Lun, K.C.; Lee, Y.N.; Tay, J. Virtual Reality for Relearning Daily Living Skills. *Int. J. Med. Inform.* **2000**, *60*, 255–261. [CrossRef] [PubMed]
18. Madhavan, K.; Kolcun, J.P.G.; Chieng, L.O.; Wang, M.Y. Augmented-Reality Integrated Robotics in Neurosurgery: Are We There Yet? *Neurosurg. Focus* **2017**, *42*, E3. [CrossRef] [PubMed]
19. Mishra, R.; Narayanan, M.D.K.; Umana, G.E.; Montemurro, N.; Chaurasia, B.; Deora, H. Virtual Reality in Neurosurgery: Beyond Neurosurgical Planning. *Int. J. Environ. Res. Public Health* **2022**, *19*, 1719. [CrossRef]
20. Abhari, K.; Baxter, J.S.H.; Chen, E.C.S.; Khan, A.R.; Peters, T.M.; De Ribaupierre, S.; Eagleson, R. Training for Planning Tumour Resection: Augmented Reality and Human Factors. *IEEE Trans. Biomed. Eng.* **2015**, *62*, 1466–1477. [CrossRef]
21. Cannizzaro, D.; Zaed, I.; Safa, A.; Jelmoni, A.J.M.; Composto, A.; Bisoglio, A.; Schmeizer, K.; Becker, A.C.; Pizzi, A.; Cardia, A.; et al. Augmented Reality in Neurosurgery, State of Art and Future Projections. A Systematic Review. *Front. Surg.* **2022**, *9*, 864792. [CrossRef] [PubMed]
22. Gasco, J.; Holbrook, T.J.; Patel, A.; Smith, A.; Paulson, D.; Muns, A.; Desai, S.; Moisi, M.; Kuo, Y.-F.; Macdonald, B.; et al. Neurosurgery Simulation in Residency Training: Feasibility, Cost, and Educational Benefit. *Neurosurgery* **2013**, *73*, S39–S45. [CrossRef] [PubMed]

23. Joseph, F.J.; Weber, S.; Raabe, A.; Bervini, D. Neurosurgical Simulator for Training Aneurysm Microsurgery—A User Suitability Study Involving Neurosurgeons and Residents. *Acta Neurochir.* **2020**, *162*, 2313–2321. [CrossRef] [PubMed]
24. Jensen, M.A.; Bhandarkar, A.R.; Riviere-Cazaux, C.; Bauman, M.M.J.; Wang, K.; Carlstrom, L.P.; Graffeo, C.S.; Spinner, R.J. The Early Bird Gets the Worm: Introducing Medical Students to Microsurgical Technique via a Low-Cost, User-Friendly, Reusable Simulation System. *World Neurosurg.* **2022**, *167*, 89–94. [CrossRef] [PubMed]
25. Robertson, F.C.; Stapleton, C.J.; Coumans, J.-V.C.E.; Nicolosi, F.; Vooijs, M.; Blitz, S.; Guerrini, F.; Spena, G.; Giussani, C.; Zoia, C.; et al. Applying Objective Metrics to Neurosurgical Skill Development with Simulation and Spaced Repetition Learning. *J. Neurosurg.* **2023**, *139*, 1092–1100. [CrossRef]
26. Dewan, M.C.; Rattani, A.; Fieggen, G.; Arraez, M.A.; Servadei, F.; Boop, F.A.; Johnson, W.D.; Warf, B.C.; Park, K.B. Global Neurosurgery: The Current Capacity and Deficit in the Provision of Essential Neurosurgical Care. Executive Summary of the Global Neurosurgery Initiative at the Program in Global Surgery and Social Change. *J. Neurosurg.* **2018**, *130*, 1055–1064. [CrossRef] [PubMed]
27. Dada, O.E.; Ooi, S.Z.Y.; Bukenya, G.W.; Kenfack, Y.J.; Le, C.; Ohonba, E.; Adeyemo, E.; Narain, K.; Awad, A.K.; Barrie, U.; et al. Evaluating the Impact of Neurosurgical Rotation Experience in Africa on the Interest and Perception of Medical Students Towards a Career in Neurosurgery: A Continental, Multi-Centre, Cross-Sectional Study. *Front. Surg.* **2022**, *9*, 766325. [CrossRef] [PubMed]
28. Menna, G.; Kolias, A.; Esene, I.N.; Barthélemy, E.J.; Hoz, S.; Laeke, T.; Veiga Silva, A.C.; Longo-Calderón, G.M.; Baticulon, R.E.; Zabala, J.P.; et al. Reducing the Gap in Neurosurgical Education in LMICs: A Report of a Non-Profit Educational Program. *World Neurosurg.* **2024**, *182*, e792–e797. [CrossRef]

brain sciences

MDPI

Article

Comparative Analysis on Vestibular Schwannoma Surgery with and without Intraoperative Fluorescein Sodium Enhancement

Amer A. Alomari [1,2], Sadeen Sameer Eid [3], Flavia Fraschetti [1], Silvia Michelini [4] and Luciano Mastronardi [1,*]

1 Department of Neurosurgery, San Filippo Neri Hospital/ASLRoma1, 00135 Rome, Italy; aaalomari07@med.just.edu.jo (A.A.A.); flavia.fraschetti@gmail.com (F.F.)
2 Division of Neurosurgery, Department of Special Surgery, Faculty of Medicine, Mutah University, Al-Karak 61710, Jordan
3 Faculty of Medicine, Jordan University of Science and Technology, Irbid 22110, Jordan; sseid19@med.just.edu.jo
4 Department of Neurosurgery, University of Tor Vergata, 00133 Rome, Italy; silviamichelini1992@gmail.com
* Correspondence: mastronardinch@gmail.com; Tel.: +39-06-60102318

Abstract: Background: Vestibular schwannoma (VS), also known as acoustic neuroma, is a benign, well-encapsulated, and slow-growing tumor that originates from Schwann cells, which form the myelin sheath around the vestibulocochlear nerve (VIII cranial nerve). The surgical treatment of this condition presents a challenging task for surgeons, as the tumor's location and size make it difficult to remove without causing damage to the surrounding structures. In recent years, fluorescein sodium (FS) has been proposed as a tool to enhance surgical outcomes in VS surgery. This essay will provide an analytical comparison of the use of FS in VS surgery, evaluating its benefits and limitations and comparing surgical outcomes with and without FS-assisted surgery. Methods: In a retrospective study conducted at San Filippo Neri Hospital, we examined VS cases that were operated on between January 2017 and December 2023. The patients were divided into two groups: group A, which consisted of patients who underwent surgery without the use of FS until January 2020 (102 cases), and group B, which included patients who underwent surgery with FS after January 2020 (55 cases). All operations were performed using the retrosigmoid approach, and tumor size was classified according to the Koos, et al. classification system. The extent of surgical removal was evaluated using both the intraoperative surgeon's opinion and postoperative MRI imaging. Preoperatively and postoperatively, facial nerve function and hearing were assessed. In group B, FS was used to assist the surgical procedures, which were performed using a surgical microscope equipped with an integrated fluorescein filter. Postoperative clinical and MRI controls were performed at six months and annually, with no patients lost to follow-up. Results: This study investigated the impact of intraoperative fluorescein exposure on tumor resection and clinical outcomes in patients with VS. The study found a statistically significant difference in the tumor resection rates between patients who received fluorescein intraoperatively ($p = 0.037$). Further analyses using the Koos classification system revealed a significant effect of fluorescein exposure, particularly in the Koos 3 subgroup ($p = 0.001$). Notably, no significant differences were observed in hearing loss or facial nerve function between the two groups. A Spearman correlation analysis revealed a positive correlation between tumor size and Koos, age, and size, but no significant correlation was found between facial nerve function tests. Conclusions: FS-assisted surgery for VS may potentially enhance tumor resection, allowing for more comprehensive tumor removal.

Keywords: vestibular schwannoma; acoustic neuroma; fluorescein sodium; facial nerve function

1. Introduction

According to the World Health Organization (WHO), schwannomas are classified as grade I benign tumors, and they typically occur as solitary tumors in approximately 90% of cases. However, in some instances, multiple tumors can develop in the same individual, which can lead to syndromic associations such as neurofibromatosis type 2 (NF2), schwannomatosis, and Carney complex [1–3]. Among all nerve sheath tumors, schwannomas are the most common, with approximately 89% of them originating from the vestibular nerve. Notably, about 60% of all schwannomas are actually vestibular schwannomas (VSs) [4].

VS, also known as acoustic neuroma, is a benign, encapsulated, and slow-growing tumor that originates from Schwann cells, which form the myelin sheath around the vestibulocochlear nerve (VIII cranial nerve). These tumors account for approximately 8% of all intracranial tumors, and most patients diagnosed are in their fourth and sixth decades of life. The condition affects both men and women equally [5,6]. A patient's clinical presentation may include symptoms such as reduced hearing, tinnitus, and imbalance, as well as facial nerve palsy, which is rare and may occur later in the course of the disease [7].

The treatment for VS involves a personalized approach, with the ultimate goal of addressing the unique needs and circumstances of each patient [8]. For small, asymptomatic schwannomas, a conservative approach involving observation with serial imaging and surgery only when the tumor shows growth may be the most appropriate option [9]. Conversely, surgery may be considered if the lesion is growing or causing symptoms. The decision on the treatment strategy depends on several factors, including the patient's age, health history, hearing status, tumor size, and presence of NF2 [8].

Fluorescein sodium (FS) is a fluorescent dye that has been employed in various medical procedures, including ophthalmology, neurosurgery, and cardiology [10,11]. In VS surgery, FS is administered intravenously before surgery and accumulates in the tumor's blood vessels. Under a specialized microscope filter (yellow 560), the tumor's blood vessels glow, allowing the surgeon to differentiate between the tumor and surrounding structures and remove the tumor with greater precision [12].

Although there is a lack of research on the effects of FS in VS resection surgery, this study provides an opportunity to investigate this research gap. The primary objective of this study was to compare the surgical outcomes of FS-assisted surgery (FSAS) and non-FS-assisted surgery in terms of the extent of removal, facial nerve function, and hearing levels. By filling this knowledge gap, our study aims to provide important insights into the benefits of FSAS in achieving successful VS operations and address the safety profile and dosage for the use of intravenous FS in neurosurgical practice for VS surgery.

2. Materials and Methods

2.1. Study Design

We retrospectively reviewed all VS cases that underwent surgery by the last author (LM) at San Filippo Neri Community Hospital of Rome between January 2017 and December 2023.

We divided the patients into two groups: group A, comprising 102 patients who underwent surgery between January 2017 and February 2020 and were operated on without FS, and group B, comprising 55 patients who underwent surgery between February 2020 and December 2023 and were operated on with the use of FSAS.

All patients underwent magnetic resonance imaging (MRI) scans, including both non-contrast and gadolinium-contrast imaging, within 1 month prior to admission. Tumor measurements were taken in three dimensions, based on the axial and coronal MRI section planes, and the maximum diameter in centimeters was estimated. The tumors were then classified according to the Koos et al. [13] classification system.

The extent of surgical removal was classified as follows: total (100%), near-total (>95%), subtotal (95–90%), and partial (<90%). The extent of removal was evaluated intraoperatively and using postoperative gadolinium-enhanced MRI, which was performed 24–48 h after surgery.

Facial nerve (N VII) function was evaluated preoperatively using the House-Brackmann (HB) grading system [14]. Additionally, facial nerve function was assessed immediately postoperatively and 6 months after follow-up.

The preoperative audio-vestibular evaluation included pure-tone audiometry and speech audiometry. The hearing levels were graded according to the American Academy of Otolaryngology-Head and Neck Surgery (AAO-HNS) classification system [15]. Classes A and B were considered socially useful hearing, while hearing preservation corresponded to classes A, B, and C, with class C indicating a level of hearing less than 50% that was not socially useful. Hearing preservation was attempted only in patients who had a preoperative hearing level classified as A or B.

2.2. Surgical Technique

All operations (for both groups) were performed using the retrosigmoid approach in the lateral Fukushima position with the use of intraoperative neuromonitoring. Neuronavigation was not used in any case (the retrosigmoid approach was performed with the use of anatomical landmarks starting with skin incision—the superior and inferior nuchal lines, then craniotomy—the digastric groove, asterion, and the opening of the internal auditory canal—the suprameatal tubercle and Tübingen line, and the tumor was debulked from inside until the capsule became liable to move and remove).

All patients in group B received FS at a standard dose of 5 mg/kg at the time of skin incision. All operations were performed using a surgical microscope with an integrated fluorescein filter, specifically the Leica ARveo ® FL560 model (Leica Microsystems, Wetzar and Mannheim, Germany), which enabled the observation of fluorophores with an excitation range of 460–500 nm. This allowed for the simultaneous viewing of non-fluorescent tissue in a natural color and fluorescent tissue in a bright yellowish-green color.

2.3. Clinical Follow Up

Clinical and radiological follow-ups were scheduled for six months after the operation and then annually, with the final date set for 15 December 2023.

The facial nerve outcomes were categorized according to the House-Brackmann grading system, which ranges from grade I to grade VI. The hearing level was classified according to the American Academy of Otolaryngology-Head and Neck Surgery (AAO-HNS) classification system, which ranges from A to D. Notably, there were no patients lost to follow-up. However, ten patients underwent surgery less than six months prior to the scheduled follow-up time and, therefore, did not meet the required follow up period. To address this issue, missing data values were substituted with median values that had been calculated for each variable.

2.4. Statistical Analysis

The statistical analysis was conducted using SPSS software (version 25), and p-values < 0.05 were considered significant, while p-values $\geq$ 0.05 were considered non-significant (NS).

The use of median imputation to eliminate and handle missing data allowed for a robust study, thereby avoiding any bias in interpreting the findings. All statistical tests and analyses were performed on the imputed dataset to ensure that all findings were valid.

3. Illustrative Cases

3.1. Case Number 1

A 34-year-old female patient, previously unremarkable in her medical and surgical history, presented with symptoms of ataxia and hearing impairment. Upon physical examination, the patient's condition was found to be intact, except for the ataxia. MRI revealed a left-sided VS, classified as Koos grade 3. Based on the patient's condition, surgical excision was planned and performed with the intraoperative assistance of FS, as depicted in Figure 1. Notably, under the microscope filter, the tumor was observed to be yellowish-green in color, while the facial nerve remained normal in its white color. Additionally, a postoperative MRI control was performed within 24–48 h to assess the patient's outcome.

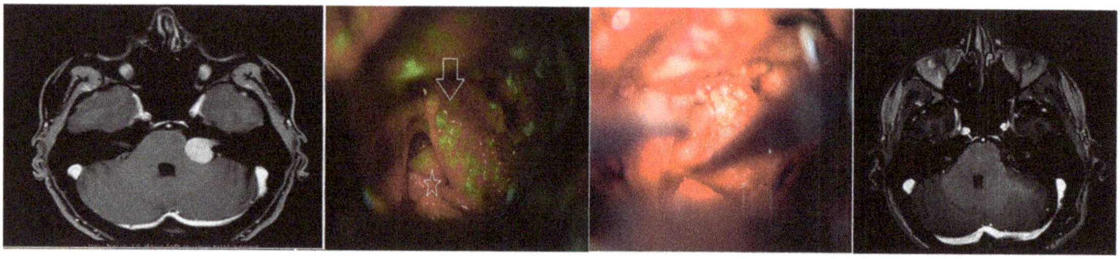

Figure 1. This figure illustrates a preoperative MRI with contrast, as well as intraoperative views of the tumor, which is depicted in yellow-green color under the filter (indicated by the arrow). The facial nerve is white (star). The figure also includes a normal microscopic view without a filter and a postoperative control MRI for comparison.

3.2. *Case Number 2*

A 60-year-old female patient with a history of hypertension presented with a 5-year decline in hearing due to a small VS. Despite her initial hearing loss, the VS exhibited further growth over the past year with further hearing impairment. Initially, the patient refused radiation therapy and instead opted for observation and potential surgical intervention. After being presented with options for management (observation, radiotherapy, and surgical excision), she elected to undergo surgical excision. The patient's preoperative, intraoperative, and postoperative images are displayed in Figure 2. Postoperatively, she experienced HB grade 2 facial weakness, which resolved after one week. At three-month follow-up, her facial nerve function had returned to normal.

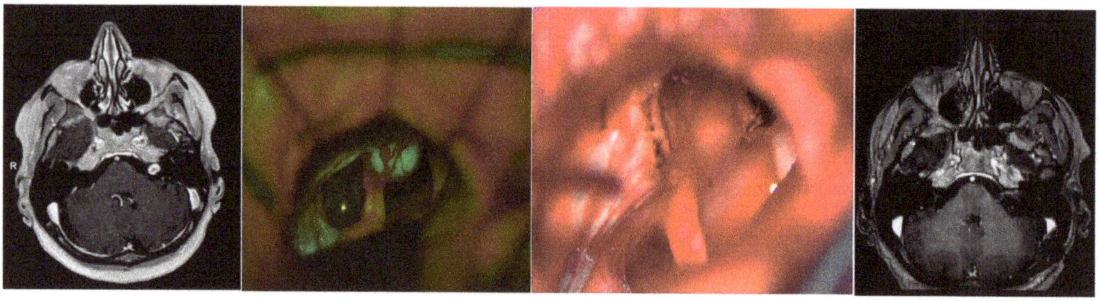

Figure 2. This figure illustrates an MRI study of a small VS as well as intraoperative imaging with a yellow 560 filter. The image shows the tumor arising from the internal auditory canal, enhancing yellowish-green color, and the non affected nerve appears white. The image on the right depicts the final result after opening the canal and removing the tumor, and the postoperative MRI control images are also included.

3.3. *Case Number 3*

In the Supplementary Materials you can find a short intraoperative video for FS-assisted surgery case.

4. Results

The total number of patients included in this study was 157 patients.

This study comprised two groups: group A, comprising 102 patients (63 females and 39 males) with no intraoperative FS use, including 56 patients who had tumors on the right side, and the mean tumor size was 2.64 cm. Group B, comprising 55 patients (32 females and 23 males), received intraoperative FS, including 29 patients who had tumors on the right side, and the mean tumor size was 2.34 cm. The observed side effects of FS were one case of a moderate reaction (extravasation and skin eruption), which was 1.8%, and two cases of mild reactions (nausea and vomiting), which was 3.6%.

The majority of patients in both cohorts with and without intraoperative FS rated their Koos grade as 2, with frequencies of 36.3% and 49.1%, respectively.

Regarding the extent of removal, most patients who did not receive intraoperative FS underwent complete resections in 74.5% of cases, followed by near-total resections in 19.6% of cases, while only a small percentage (5.9%) had subtotal resections.

The total resection rate was 56.4% in patients treated with FSAS, while near-total resections accounted for 40% of cases, resulting in a subtotal resection rate of 3.6%.

Tables 1 and 2 provide a summary of the clinical and radiological findings for each group.

Table 1. Analysis of age and tumor size for both groups.

Fluoresceine		Age	Size
No	Mean	50.12	2.642
	Number	102	102
	Standard Deviation	13.522	0.935
Yes	Mean	51.36	2.340
	Number	55	55
	Standard Deviation	10.94	0.837
Total	Mean	50.55	2.536
	Number	157	157
	Standard Deviation	12.655	0.911

Table 2. Clinical and radiological characteristics for both groups in this study.

Fluoresceine		Sex		Koos				Removal Extent		
		M	F	1	2	3	4	T	NT	ST
No	Frequency	39	63	1	37	35	29	76	20	6
	Percent	38.2	61.8	1	36.3	34.3	28.4	74.5	19.6	5.9
Yes	Frequency	23	32	3	27	15	10	31	22	2
	Percent	41.8	58.2	5.5	49.1	27.3	18.2	56.4	40	3.6

T: total resection, NT: near-total resection, ST: subtotal resection.

A crosstabulation analysis was conducted to examine the relationship between the preoperative hearing loss (PRE-HL) assessment and postoperative hearing loss (POST-HL) assessment, as presented in Tables 3 and 4.

Table 3. Fluoresceine PRE-HL crosstabulation count.

		PRE-HL				Total
		A	B	C	D	
Fluoresceine	No	7	21	47	27	102
	Yes	1	20	24	10	55
Total		8	41	71	37	157

Table 4. Fluoresceine POST-HL crosstabulation count.

		POST-HL					Total
		A	B	C	Missing	D	
Fluoresceine	No	4	11	33	0	54	102
	Yes	1	7	21	10	16	55
Total		5	18	54	10	70	157

To investigate whether there was a difference in the tumor resection degree between the patients who received FS and those who did not, we performed a Mann–Whitney test. The resulting p-value of 0.037 indicated statistical significance, suggesting a significant difference in the extent of the removal rates between the two groups, as shown in Table 5. Specifically, the mean rank for patients receiving fluorescein was 87.42, compared to 74.42 for those who did not receive fluorescein. The Z-value of −2.09, which reflects a mild observed difference in accordance with Cohen's 1992 standards for effect size interpretation, suggests that this difference is considered effective.

Table 5. Mann–Whitney test.

	Removal Extent	Early HB	Post HL	Late HB
Mann–Whitney U	2342.000	2623.000	2410.000	2668.500
Wilcoxon W	7595.000	4163.000	3950.000	7921.500
Z	−2.090	−0.797	−1.559	−0.765
Asymp. Sig. (2-tailed)	**0.037**	0.425	0.119	0.444

Significant differences in tumor resection rates were observed between the patients with and without fluorescein (p = 0.037), However, fluorescein showed no significant impact on hearing loss or facial nerve function, with all p-values exceeding 0.05.

After finding a statistically significant correlation between sodium fluorescein administration and tumor extension excision, we performed further analyses by categorizing patients according to the Koos classification. We then conducted separate Mann–Whitney tests within each Koos category to examine the specific effect of fluorescein on different clinical stages. Notably, we obtained a p-value of 0.001 for the Koos 3 group, indicating that fluorescein administration had a significant effect on this specific subgroup. The mean rank results showed that patients who received fluorescein had a mean rank of 33.7, compared to 21.9 for those who did not receive fluorescein.

Additionally, we used the Mann–Whitney test to investigate the effect of fluorescein administration on hearing loss and facial nerve function. The results showed no statistically significant difference between the patients who received fluorescein and those who did not in terms of either hearing loss or facial nerve function. The p-values for all three outcomes were non-significant, exceeding the 0.05 significance threshold, indicating a lack of significance, as shown in Table 5.

A Spearman's correlation analysis was employed to examine the relationship between tumor removal extension and various parameters, including Koos, age, tumor size, postoperative assessment of hearing loss, and early and late assessments of facial nerve function, as presented in Table 6.

Table 6. Results of the Spearman's correlation analysis.

		Koos	Age	Size	Post HL	Late HB	Early HB
Removal	Correlation Coefficient	0.270	0.167	0.306	0.230	0.123	0.109
	Sig. (2-tailed)	0.001	0.037	0.000	0.004	0.126	0.175
	Number	157	157	157	157	157	157

Positive correlations between the degree of extensions to Koos, age, size, and hearing loss assessment after surgical procedures. No statistically significant correlation was found between the early and late assessments of facial nerve function.

5. Discussion

5.1. Management of Vestibular Schwannoma

VS treatment options are diverse and may include observation, surgical resection, and radiation therapy. Each option is tailored to individual patient circumstances, considering factors such as age, overall health, tumor size, symptoms, growth rate, and other relevant characteristics. Treatment options can be adjusted as needed based on changes in patient status, such as symptom progression or growth rate. Surgical resection techniques are several, which may include retrosigmoid, translabyrinthine, subtemporal approaches, or combinations of these approaches, depending on factors such as tumor size, surgeon expertise, and intracanalicular extension.

Resection surgeries aiming for complete resection have been shown to have the most beneficial outcomes, with significantly better short-term and long-term results compared to incomplete tumor removal. Notably, patients who undergo complete resection experience lower rates of recurrence and higher rates of successful resection [16]. A comprehensive review of 1000 VS resections reported a remarkable 98% complete resection rate, as well as a 68% hearing preservation rate. Additionally, the mortality rate associated with these surgeries was remarkably low, at just 1% [17]. Notably, the risk of local recurrence after a complete resection is extremely low, ranging from 0% to 2%. In contrast, if only the partial removal of the tumor is possible, the incidence of tumor recurrence is significantly higher, at approximately 30% [17]. Despite advances in surgical techniques, the complete resection of VS may still be challenging due to their adhesion to surrounding nerves or brain structures, which can increase the risk of incomplete resection or damage to normal tissues [18]. This uncertainty has led to questions about the potential benefits of integrating neural-guided techniques into intracranial tumor resection, which could potentially improve gross total resection while protecting normal vital tissues and enhancing patient outcomes.

5.2. Application of Fluorescein Sodium

The first application of fluoresceine in neurosurgery was in 1948 by Moore et al. [19], where it was used for the identification of several types of brain tumors, and recently it has been used more in high-grade gliomas [20], meningiomas [21], skull base tumors [10], less common VS [12], and peripheral schwannomas [22].

5.3. Safety of Fluorescein Sodium

FS is now widely used in neurosurgery for oncology and neurovascular purposes. It has been applied for many years in general surgery, gastroenterology, and mainly in ophthalmology with a safe profile [23].

Yannuzzi et al. [23] classified the adverse reactions of the intravenous use of FS based on the duration, need for intervention, and final outcome into mild, moderate, or severe reactions. The severe reactions—including cardiovascular, respiratory, neurological, or death—were extremely rarely reported, and in our series, we did not report any severe reactions. Moderate reactions included the development of skin eruption, syncope, local tissue necrosis, thrombophlebitis, pyrexia, and nerve palsy. The development of skin eruption represented the most common of the moderate reactions, and we had one case that developed skin eruption that was treated with a regular dressing and oral antihistamine. Mild reactions represented the most common reactions to FS, represented by nausea and vomiting, extravasation, inadvertent intraarterial injection, sneezing, and pruritis. In our series, we had two cases that developed nausea and vomiting; it was for one to two days and then resolved spontaneously, and another case that had an extravasation, which was treated conservatively with arm raises and exercise.

Restelli et al. [24] conducted a comprehensive neurosurgical literature review on the safety of FS and found that FS was shown to be extremely safe in neurosurgery, including oncological and neurovascular cases, even at high doses.

5.4. Dosage of Fluorescein Sodium

FS has been used in neurosurgery at various stages, where it was previously used at large dosages (40 mg/kg) for a low-grade glioma or a re-dose was used to promote tumor enhancement under a microscope, with the main reason being a lack of fitted specific filters on surgical microscopes [20,25,26]. According to recent extensive research [24], the current tendency is to utilize lower doses (about 5 mg/kg) due to the availability of microscopes with wavelength-specific filters for FS. In our series, we employed a fixed dosage and timing of 5 mg/kg at the time of skin incision.

5.5. Mechanism of Enhancement

Yan Xiang et al. [27] found that sodium fluoresceine-assisted surgery is effective for high-grade glioma surgery since FS presence is directly related to the breakdown of the blood-brain barrier (BBB) in the tumor. On the counterpart, VSs are benign and often hypervascular tumors, and the presence of FS could be explained by the pathological blood vessels of the tumor rather than the breakdown of the BBB. Therefore, FS can be used to aid in the recognition of the facial and cochlear nerves from the tumor, potentially assisting the surgeon in anatomical preservation for the normal nerves with a greater extent of resection, as we found from our comparison results.

5.6. Maximal Safe Resection

The existing literature consistently highlights a notable trend: incomplete resection for patients with VS is linked to a higher incidence of progression or regrowth compared to patients who underwent total resection [28]. Based on the current knowledge, the present study researched a narrow spectrum, studying the possibility of sodium fluorescein's impact on VS resection and follow-up clinical outcomes. Our goal was to focus on this particular aspect and create a comprehensive discussion on the greater completeness of tumor removal, which may increase the various gain rates in the administration of FS in patients with VS. This specific research is in line with the final objective, which is to improve treatment options and enhance the outcomes of patients in the context of VS management.

Fluorescein-guided surgery allows for the more precise identification of tumor borderlines from the adjacent structures (the facial nerve, trigeminal nerve, lower cranial nerves, and brainstem), simplifying a more radical resection. The data of our study shows a significant difference in tumor removal between the patients who received fluorescein and those who did not, with the greatest differences observed among the patients categorized as Koos 3. As a result, the operation may have been performed more radically using fluorescein to be sure of the complete removal of the tumor while the important structures are preserved. The results endorse the use of fluorescein as a targeted adjunct in VS microsurgery, which in turn opens the door for the further development of surgical techniques.

5.7. Hearing Level

The positive and significant correlation between tumor resection and hearing loss in patients undergoing surgery is also of particular interest. This implies that more extensive tumor removal comes at the cost of more destruction of the auditory structures, thus producing worse hearing outcomes. This might happen due to the close adhesion of the tumor to the vital auditory structures like the cochlear nerve during operation [29,30]. Other studies have suggested that the surgical technique can preserve hearing function, especially in smaller tumors [30,31].

5.8. Facial Nerve

The results of our research demonstrate no statistically significant correlation between the extent of tumor resection and facial nerve function. This is consistent with findings from many other studies [32,33]. This finding indicates that the use of fluorescein does not lead to improved facial motor function outcomes, especially when looked at from the perspective of VS removal. Other factors that may turn out to be an important determinant of facial nerve function outcomes include the tumor size, adherence of the tumor to the nerve, hypervascularized tumors, facial nerve function before the operation, and age of the patient [32–34].

5.9. Limitations

Although this study has provided us with some invaluable knowledge, some limitations have to be noted. The limitations associated with this study may include the sample size of a known cohort and the nature of a retrospective analysis, which may bring about some biases. Future studies should be directed at filling these gaps since fluorescein can only be considered as having the potential to cause changes in the tumor resection results, and this may have a clinical impact.

5.10. Summary

Our cohort study provides valuable insights into the role of sodium fluorescein in VS surgery, particularly regarding its impact on the extent of resection and postoperative functional outcomes for facial and cochlear nerves. Notably, FS was found to be safe and well-tolerated at a dose of 5 mg/kg, with only mild to moderate adverse reactions reported. However, further research is needed to fully assess the safety of FS in neurosurgery practice, including the optimal timing and dosing, as well as the possibility of redosing if necessary.

6. Conclusions

FS-assisted surgery for VS may have a substantial influence on the extent of tumor resection, with no discernible effects on postoperative hearing and facial nerve function. Moreover, FS is deemed safe for use in VS surgery.

Supplementary Materials: The following supporting information can be downloaded at: https://www.mdpi.com/article/10.3390/brainsci14060571/s1. This video shows a patient with a left VS, classified as Koos 3, undergoing surgery using intraoperative neuromonitoring in the lateral Fukushima position via the retrosigmoid approach. The surgical approach begins by carefully checking the facial nerve position, followed by opening of the capsule using a hand-held Thulium laser. Next, the tumor is debulked intracapsular to make it suitable for detachment from surrounding tissue. As part of the procedure, the facial nerve is identified and verified using a filtered lens (FL560), which allows us to visualize the nerve in its normal white color and distinguish it from the tumor. The tumor is then glowing yellowish-green, while the capsule is dark and non-enhancing. This allows for careful dissection of the tumor from the nerve, minimizing potential injury or traction. Finally, postoperative control MRI is shown at the end of the video to confirm successful tumor resection. This video demonstrates a successful application of fluorescein-assisted surgery for VS resection, highlighting the potential benefits of this technique for improved patient outcomes.

Author Contributions: A.A.A.: data extraction, data analysis, study conception, manuscript writing. S.S.E.: data extraction, statistical analysis, literature analysis, manuscript writing. F.F.: data extraction, data analysis, literature analysis. S.M.: resources. L.M.: study design, study conception, data extraction, data analysis, manuscript writing, and reviewing. All authors have read and agreed to the published version of the manuscript.

Funding: This research received no external funding.

Institutional Review Board Statement: The study involved human participants; therefore, it has been reviewed and approved by the local ethics committee of the hospital. Written consent for the scientific treatment of personal data was obtained from all patients before surgery. No potentially identifiable human images or data are presented in this study. All procedures performed in this study were in accordance with the ethical standards of the internal institutional ethics committee: "Comitato Etico Lazio 1" Members of ASLRoma1: Dr. Marco Tubaro, Dr. Teresa Calamia, Dr. Francesco Meo (SFN02/2022, 31 January 2022).

Informed Consent Statement: Written consent was obtained from all patients included in the study.

Data Availability Statement: The data are only available upon request from the last author due to restrictions, privacy, legal, or ethical reasons.

Conflicts of Interest: The authors declare no conflicts of interest.

References

1. Lee, S.-U.; Bae, Y.J.; Kim, H.-J.; Choi, J.-Y.; Song, J.-J.; Choi, B.Y.; Koo, J.-W.; Kim, J.-S. Intralabyrinthine schwannoma: Distinct features for differential diagnosis. *Front. Neurol.* **2019**, *10*, 750. [CrossRef] [PubMed]
2. Coy, S.; Rashid, R.; Stemmer-Rachamimov, A.; Santagata, S. Correction to: An update on the CNS manifestations of neurofibromatosis type 2. *Acta Neuropathol.* **2020**, *139*, 667. [CrossRef] [PubMed]
3. Kamilaris, C.D.; Faucz, F.R.; Voutetakis, A.; Stratakis, C.A. Carney complex. *Exp. Clin. Endocrinol. Diabetes* **2019**, *127*, 156–164. [CrossRef] [PubMed]

4. Propp, J.M.; McCarthy, B.J.; Davis, F.G.; Preston-Martin, S. Descriptive epidemiology of vestibular schwannomas. *Neuro-oncology* **2006**, *8*, 1–11. [CrossRef] [PubMed]
5. Pandrangi, V.C.; Han, A.Y.; Alonso, J.E.; Peng, K.A.; John, M.A.S. An update on epidemiology and management trends of vestibular schwannomas. *Otol. Neurotol.* **2020**, *41*, 411–417. [CrossRef]
6. Reznitsky, M.; Petersen MM, B.S.; West, N.; Stangerup, S.E.; Cayé-Thomasen, P. Epidemiology and diagnostic characteristics of vestibular schwannomas—Does gender matter? *Otol. Neurotol.* **2020**, *41*, e1372–e1378. [CrossRef] [PubMed]
7. Matthies, C.; Samii, M. Management of 1000 vestibular schwannomas (acoustic neuromas): Clinical presentation. *Neurosurgery* **1997**, *40*, 1–10.
8. Nikolopoulos, T.P.; Fortnum, H.; O'Donoghue, G.; Baguley, D. Acoustic neuroma growth: A systematic review of the evidence. *Otol. Neurotol.* **2010**, *31*, 478–485. [CrossRef]
9. Suryanarayanan, R.; Ramsden, R.T.; Saeed, S.R.; Aggarwal, R.; King, A.T.; Rutherford, S.A.; Evans, D.G.; Gillespie, J.E. Vestibular schwannoma: Role of conservative management. *J. Laryngol. Otol.* **2010**, *124*, 251–257. [CrossRef]
10. Da Silva, C.E.; da Silva, J.L.B.; da Silva, V.D. Use of sodium fluorescein in skull base tumors. *Surg. Neurol. Int.* **2010**, *1*, 70. [CrossRef]
11. Hayreh, S.S. Recent advances in fluorescein fundus angiography. *Br. J. Ophthalmol.* **1974**, *58*, 391. [CrossRef] [PubMed]
12. Misra, B.K.; Jha, A.K. Potential utility of sodium fluorescein can distinguish tumor from cranial nerves in vestibular schwannoma surgery. *Neurol. India* **2021**, *69*, 1087–1088. [CrossRef]
13. Koos, W.T.; Day, J.D.; Matula, C.; Levy, D.I. Neurotopographic considerations in the microsurgical treatment of small acoustic neurinomas. *J. Neurosurg.* **1998**, *88*, 506–512. [CrossRef] [PubMed]
14. House, J.W.; Brackmann, D.E. Facial nerve grading system. *Otolaryngol. Head Neck Surg.* **1985**, *93*, 146–147. [CrossRef] [PubMed]
15. Committee on Hearing and Equilibrium. Committee on Hearing and Equilibrium guidelines for the evaluation of hearing preservation in acoustic neuroma (vestibular schwannoma). *Otolaryngol. Head Neck Surg.* **1995**, *113*, 179–180. [CrossRef] [PubMed]
16. Karpinos, M.; Teh, B.S.; Zeck, O.; Carpenter, L.S.; Phan, C.; Mai, W.-Y.; Lu, H.H.; Chiu, J.K.; Butler, E.B.; Gormley, W.B. Treatment of acoustic neuroma: Stereotactic radiosurgery vs. microsurgery. *Int. J. Radiat. Oncol. Biol. Phys.* **2002**, *54*, 1410–1421. [CrossRef] [PubMed]
17. Samii, M.; Matthies, C. Management of 1000 vestibular schwannomas (acoustic neuromas): Surgical management and results with an emphasis on complications and how to avoid them. *Neurosurgery* **1997**, *40*, 11–23. [PubMed]
18. Carlson, M.L.; Link, M.J. Vestibular schwannomas. *N. Engl. J. Med.* **2021**, *384*, 1335–1348. [CrossRef] [PubMed]
19. Moore, G.E.; Peyton, W.T.; French, L.A.; Walker, W.W. The clinical use of fluorscein in neurosurgery. The localization of brain tumors. *J. Neurosurg.* **1948**, *5*, 392–398. [CrossRef] [PubMed]
20. Shinoda, J.; Yano, H.; Yoshimura, S.-I.; Okumura, A.; Kaku, Y.; Iwama, T.; Sakai, N. Fluorescence-guided resection of glioblastoma multiforme by using high-dose fluorescein sodium. *J. Neurosurg.* **2003**, *99*, 597–603. [CrossRef] [PubMed]
21. Dijkstra, B.M.; Jeltema, H.-R.; Kruijff, S.; Groen, R.J.M. The application of fluorescence techniques in meningioma surgery—A review. *Neurosurg. Rev.* **2019**, *42*, 799–809. [CrossRef] [PubMed]
22. Kalamarides, M.; Bernat, I.; Peyre, M. Extracapsular dissection in peripheral nerve schwannoma surgery using bright light and fluorescein sodium visualization: Case series. *Acta Neurochir.* **2019**, *161*, 2447–2452. [CrossRef] [PubMed]
23. Yannuzzi, L.A.; Rohrer, K.T.; Tindel, L.J.; Sobel, R.S.; Costanza, M.A.; Shields, W.; Zang, E. Fluorescein angiography complication survey. *Ophthalmology* **1986**, *93*, 611–617. [CrossRef] [PubMed]
24. Restelli, F.; Mathis, A.M.; Höhne, J.; Mazzapicchi, E.; Acerbi, F.; Pollo, B.; Quint, K. Confocal laser imaging in neurosurgery: A comprehensive review of sodium fluorescein-based CONVIVO preclinical and clinical applications. *Front. Oncol.* **2022**, *12*, 998384. [CrossRef] [PubMed]
25. Abramov, I.; Dru, A.B.; Belykh, E.; Park, M.T.; Bardonova, L.; Preul, M.C. Redosing of fluorescein sodium improves image interpretation during intraoperative ex vivo confocal laser endomicroscopy of brain tumors. *Front. Oncol.* **2021**, *11*, 668661. [CrossRef] [PubMed]
26. Belykh, E.; Onaka, N.R.; Zhao, X.; Abramov, I.; Eschbacher, J.M.; Nakaji, P.; Preul, M.C. High-dose fluorescein reveals unusual confocal endomicroscope imaging of low-grade glioma. *Front. Neurol.* **2021**, *12*, 668656. [CrossRef] [PubMed]
27. Xiang, Y.; Zhu, X.-P.; Zhao, J.-N.; Huang, G.-H.; Tang, J.-H.; Chen, H.-R.; Du, L.; Zhang, D.; Tang, X.-F.; Yang, H.; et al. Blood-brain barrier disruption, sodium fluorescein, and fluorescence-guided surgery of gliomas. *Br. J. Neurosurg.* **2018**, *32*, 141–148. [CrossRef] [PubMed]
28. Bloch, D.C.; Oghalai, J.S.; Jackler, R.K.; Osofsky, M.; Pitts, L.H. The fate of the tumor remnant after less-than-complete acoustic neuroma resection. *Otolaryngol. Head Neck Surg.* **2004**, *130*, 104–112. [CrossRef] [PubMed]
29. Gan, J.; Zhang, Y.; Wu, J.; Lei, D.; Zhang, F.; Zhao, H.; Wang, L. Current understanding of hearing loss in sporadic vestibular schwannomas: A systematic review. *Front. Oncol.* **2021**, *11*, 687201. [CrossRef] [PubMed]
30. Ariano, M.; Franchella, S.; Tealdo, G.; Zanoletti, E. Intra-Operative Cochlear Nerve Function Monitoring in Hearing Preservation Surgery: A Systematic Review of the Literature. *Audiol. Res.* **2022**, *12*, 696–708. [CrossRef] [PubMed]
31. Concheri, S.; Deretti, A.; Tealdo, G.; Zanoletti, E. Prognostic Factors for Hearing Preservation Surgery in Small Vestibular Schwannoma. *Audiol. Res.* **2023**, *13*, 473–483. [CrossRef] [PubMed]

32. Bloch, O.; Sughrue, M.E.; Kaur, R.; Kane, A.J.; Rutkowski, M.J.; Kaur, G.; Yang, I.; Pitts, L.H.; Parsa, A.T. Factors associated with preservation of facial nerve function after surgical resection of vestibular schwannoma. *J. Neuro-Oncol.* **2011**, *102*, 281–286. [CrossRef] [PubMed]
33. Ren, Y.; MacDonald, B.V.; Tawfik, K.O.; Schwartz, M.S.; Friedman, R.A. Clinical predictors of facial nerve outcomes after surgical resection of vestibular schwannoma. *Otolaryngol. Head Neck Surg.* **2021**, *164*, 1085–1093. [CrossRef]
34. Gazia, F.; Callejo, A.; Pérez-Grau, M.; Lareo, S.; Prades, J.; Roca-Ribas, F.; Amilibia, E. Pre-and intra-operative prognostic factors of facial nerve function in cerebellopontine angle surgery. *Eur. Arch. Oto-Rhino-Laryngol.* **2023**, *280*, 1055–1062. [CrossRef] [PubMed]

brain sciences

MDPI

Review

Invasive Brain–Computer Interface for Communication: A Scoping Review

Shujhat Khan [1], Leonie Kallis [2], Harry Mee [1,3], Salim El Hadwe [1,4], Damiano Barone [1,5], Peter Hutchinson [1,6] and Angelos Kolias [1,6,*]

1 Department of Clinical Neuroscience, University of Cambridge, Cambridge CB2 1TN, UK; sk2361@cam.ac.uk (S.K.); hwjm2@medschl.cam.ac.uk (H.M.); se471@cam.ac.uk (S.E.H.); dgb36@cam.ac.uk (D.B.); pjah2@cam.ac.uk (P.H.)
2 Department of Medicine, University of Cambridge, Trinity Ln, Cambridge CB2 1TN, UK; leonie.kallis1@nhs.net
3 Department of Rehabilitation, Addenbrookes Hospital, Hills Rd., Cambridge CB2 0QQ, UK
4 Bioelectronics Laboratory, Department of Electrical Engineering, University of Cambridge, Cambridge CB2 1PZ, UK
5 Department of Neurosurgery, Houston Methodist, Houston, TX 77079, USA
6 Department of Neurosurgery, Addenbrookes Hospital, Hills Rd., Cambridge CB2 0QQ, UK
* Correspondence: ak721@cam.ac.uk

Abstract: Background: The rapid expansion of the brain–computer interface for patients with neurological deficits has garnered significant interest, and for patients, it provides an additional route where conventional rehabilitation has its limits. This has particularly been the case for patients who lose the ability to communicate. Circumventing neural injuries by recording from the intact cortex and subcortex has the potential to allow patients to communicate and restore self-expression. Discoveries over the last 10–15 years have been possible through advancements in technology, neuroscience, and computing. By examining studies involving intracranial brain–computer interfaces that aim to restore communication, we aimed to explore the advances made and explore where the technology is heading. Methods: For this scoping review, we systematically searched PubMed and OVID Embase. After processing the articles, the search yielded 41 articles that we included in this review. Results: The articles predominantly assessed patients who had either suffered from amyotrophic lateral sclerosis, cervical cord injury, or brainstem stroke, resulting in tetraplegia and, in some cases, difficulty speaking. Of the intracranial implants, ten had ALS, six had brainstem stroke, and thirteen had a spinal cord injury. Stereoelectroencephalography was also used, but the results, whilst promising, are still in their infancy. Studies involving patients who were moving cursors on a screen could improve the speed of movement by optimising the interface and utilising better decoding methods. In recent years, intracortical devices have been successfully used for accurate speech-to-text and speech-to-audio decoding in patients who are unable to speak. Conclusions: Here, we summarise the progress made by BCIs used for communication. Speech decoding directly from the cortex can provide a novel therapeutic method to restore full, embodied communication to patients suffering from tetraplegia who otherwise cannot communicate.

Keywords: brain–computer interface; brain–machine interface; BCI; neurotechnology; paralysis; ALS; stroke; spinal cord; ECoG; multielectrode array; stereoelectroencephalography

1. Introduction

Communication is a vital part of social interaction that can be impaired following conditions such as stroke, trauma, and neuromuscular diseases (NMDs). For many patients, the deprivation of communication is severely debilitating and significantly worsens the quality of life [1]. In the most severe of cases, patients can present with a profound state of paralysis, characterised by tetraplegia, cranial nerve dysfunction, and anarthria, yet with preserved cognitive function, known as the locked-in syndrome (LIS) [2]. As such, the development and implementation of functional communication systems for this population is a clinical and research priority [3].

Conventional augmentative and alternative communication (AAC) devices rely on residual motor functions to provide a partial solution. In some cases, people who retain partial motor function can use specially modified peripherals (e.g., mouse, joysticks, stylus, or button box) to access such AAC devices [4]. In other, more severe cases where minimal voluntary motor control is retained, more sophisticated methods are needed to detect more subtle movements like those of the head, eye gaze tracking and blinking, allowing people to communicate by spelling out messages. However, these devices require considerable effort and are often slow, failing to restore the natural fluidity of communication [5,6]. Brain–computer interfaces (BCIs) offer a more promising approach by directly translating neural activity into external device control, bypassing damaged motor pathways [7]. A BCI sensor can be placed at various depths away from the target location, ranging from sensors placed on the scalp known as surface electroencephalogram (EEG) to intracortical recordings where microelectrodes are inserted within target locations of cortical tissue (Figure 1). Other invasive sensors include electrocorticography (ECoG), which sits on the cortical surface but does not penetrate, and stereotactic electroencephalography (sEEG), which includes depth electrodes that are able to record from deep brain structures [8]. However, the greatest drawbacks to invasive methods are the risks of surgical complications and anaesthesia, as well as the risk of postoperative infection [9]. As such, there have been limited cases, and of those that have been explored, participants are usually those that have otherwise very poor outcomes, for which an investigational device exemption is required.

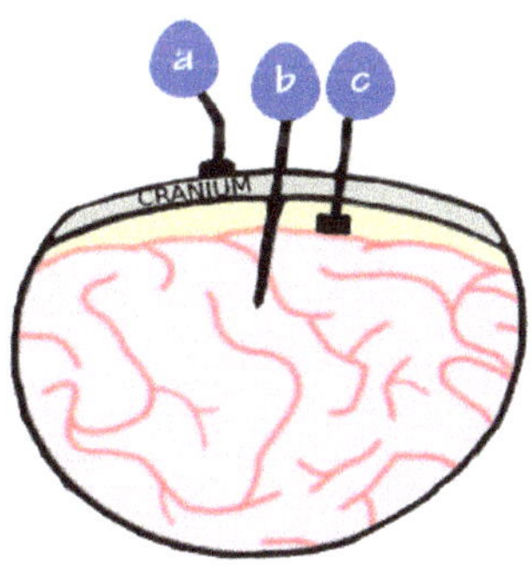

Figure 1. Image demonstrates placement of electrodes: (a) EEG that sits on top of the scalp; (b) intracortical electrodes that penetrate the cortex; (c) ECoG electrodes that are placed on the cortex but do not penetrate it.

Currently, patients with restricted communication abilities use augmentative and alternative communication devices. These include the use of neck and head movements or eye movements to be able to allow individuals to communicate by spelling out messages. However, this requires considerable effort and is slow [5]. This is where BCIs can have a major impact, as they can directly decode cortical activity and control external devices to enable more seamless communication. This scoping review provides an overview of intracortical BCIs that have been used to provide neurological rehabilitation in patients with impaired communication. Given the scale at which the field has advanced over the last decade, this review provides an update on what is currently possible in an academic setting and highlights important technical features.

2. Methods

A comprehensive literature review was conducted based on the preferred reporting items for systematic reviews and meta-analysis guidelines (PRISMA). Ovid Medline alongside PubMed were used to search for keywords and MeSh terms including "brain-computer", "neuroprosthesis", "neuroprosthetics, "intracortical", "intracortically" "brain-controlled", "brain-machine", "microelectrode array", "neuroprosthesis", "electrical neuromodulation" AND "Locked in syndrome", "locked-in-syndrome", "amyotrophic lateral sclerosis", "dysarthria", "communication", "speech", "Brain Hemorrhage", "Traumatic", "brain injury", "head injury", "Diffuse Axonal Brain Injury", "trauma", "stroke", "cerebral infarction", "cerebral hemorrhage", and "cerebral vascular accident". The full search strategy is illustrated in Figure 2.

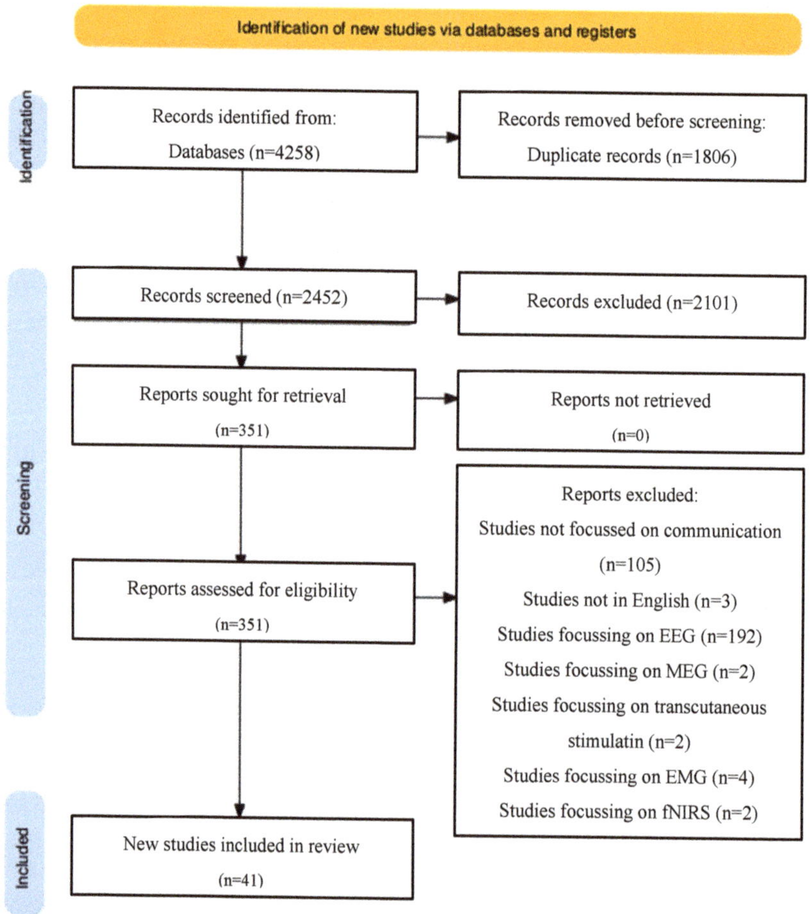

Figure 2. PRISMA reporting: preferred reporting items for systematic review and meta-analysis (PRISMA) flow chart explaining selection of articles in a step-wise manner as well as reasons for the exclusion of studies. Databases used included PubMed and Ovid Medline.

2.1. Study Types

Study types including case reports or case series were included. Due to the nature of this research, there are no large-scale published reports or randomised controlled trials (Figure 2).

2.2. Inclusion and Exclusion Criteria

All clinical studies investigating the outcomes of invasive BCIs for communication purposes were included from January 2005 to October 2024 due to the significant progress made over the last couple of decades. This included ECoG, intracortical and sEEG electrodes that enabled patients to communicate through either a digital screen or artificial voice. Additionally, only studies that were published in English were included due to resource constraints, and only human studies were considered. Whilst animal and in vitro models have been vital for the progress that has been made in this field, we wanted to focus exclusively on human studies to assess the neurotechnologies that were closest to clinical feasibility and could avoid the at-time difficult transition from animal to human testing. As such, animal or in vitro models were excluded. Review articles, non-human studies, and studies in languages other than English were excluded. Additionally, we checked reference lists of relevant publications to identify otherwise missed studies.

2.3. Research Questions

This study aimed to determine the current landscape of invasive BCIs for communication. As such, we posed a few questions:

(1) What pathology did the patient cohorts present with?
(2) How successful are intracortical BCIs in restoring communication?
(3) How many electrodes were used for implantation in intracortical devices?
(4) What task did subjects have to perform for the BCI device to convert into a method of communication?
(5) How successful are ECoG devices in restoring communication?
(6) What promise do sEEG devices have in restoring communication?
(7) Which anatomical region of the brain do BCIs target to facilitate communication?

3. Results

3.1. Patient Profile

Most of the studies occurred in the United States (US) (31/41), 5 studies were published in the Netherlands and 2 from Israel. China, Canada, and the United Kingdom each published one study (Table 1). No studies were performed on children. In studies where patients had epilepsy or movement disorders, BCIs were implanted as an opportunistic research experiment. In the remaining studies, patients either had tetraplegia or locked-in syndrome.

Table 1. Studies involving intracortical implantation for communication disorders.

Title	Year Published	Country
Measuring instability in chronic human intracortical neural recordings towards stable, long-term brain-computer interfaces [10]	2024	USA
An Accurate and Rapidly Calibrating Speech Neuroprosthesis [11]	2024	USA
A bilingual speech neuroprosthesis driven by cortical articulatory representations shared between languages [12]	2024	USA
Representation of internal speech by single neurons in human supramarginal gyrus [13]	2024	USA

Table 1. *Cont.*

Title	Year Published	Country
Online speech synthesis using a chronically implanted brain-computer interface in an individual with ALS [14]	2024	USA
Machine learning decoding of single neurons in the thalamus for speech brain-machine interfaces [15]	2024	Israel
Longevity of a Brain-Computer Interface for Amyotrophic Lateral Sclerosis [16]	2024	The Netherlands
Speech decoding from stereo-electroencephalography (sEEG) signals using advanced deep learning methods [17]	2024	UK
Stable Decoding from a Speech BCI Enables Control for an Individual with ALS without Recalibration for 3 Months [18]	2023	USA
Distributed feedforward and feedback cortical processing supports human speech production [19]	2023	USA
A high-performance neuroprosthesis for speech decoding and avatar control [20]	2023	USA
A high-performance speech neuroprosthesis [21]	2023	USA
Direct speech reconstruction from sensorimotor brain activity with optimized deep learning models [22]	2023	The Netherlands
Generalizable spelling using a speech neuroprosthesis in an individual with severe limb and vocal paralysis [23]	2022	USA
Intracranial brain-computer interface spelling using localized visual motion response [24]	2022	China
Decoding grasp and speech signals from the cortical grasp circuit in a tetraplegic human [25]	2022	USA
Machine learning algorithm for decoding multiple subthalamic spike trains for speech brain-machine interfaces [26]	2021	Israel
Real-time synthesis of imagined speech processes from minimally invasive recordings of neural activity [27]	2021	The Netherlands
Generalizable cursor click decoding using grasp-related neural transients [28]	2021	USA
Neuroprosthesis for Decoding Speech in a Paralyzed Person with Anarthria [29]	2021	USA
Home Use of a Percutaneous Wireless Intracortical Brain-Computer Interface by Individuals With Tetraplegia [30]	2021	USA
Dorsolateral prefrontal cortex-based control with an implanted brain-computer interface [31]	2020	The Netherlands
Neural ensemble dynamics in dorsal motor cortex during speech in people with paralysis [32]	2019	USA
Speech synthesis from neural decoding of spoken sentences [33]	2019	USA
Cortical control of a tablet computer by people with paralysis [34]	2018	USA
Stable long-term BCI-enabled communication in ALS and locked-in syndrome using LFP signals [35]	2018	USA
High performance communication by people with paralysis using an intracortical brain-computer interface [36]	2017	USA
Fully Implanted Brain-Computer Interface in a Locked-In Patient with ALS [37]	2016	The Netherlands
Virtual typing by people with tetraplegia using a self-calibrating intracortical brain-computer interface [38]	2015	USA
Decoding of articulatory gestures during word production using speech motor and premotor cortical activity [39]	2015	USA
Neural Point-and-Click Communication by a Person With Incomplete Locked-In Syndrome [40]	2015	USA
Real-time two-dimensional asynchronous control of a computer cursor with a single subdural electrode [41]	2012	Canada
Neural control of cursor trajectory and click by a human with tetraplegia 1000 days after implant of an intracortical microelectrode array [42]	2011	USA

Table 1. *Cont.*

Title	Year Published	Country
Using the electrocorticographic speech network to control a brain-computer interface in humans [43]	2011	USA
Control of a brain-computer interface using stereotactic depth electrodes in and adjacent to the hippocampus [44]	2011	USA
Point-and-click cursor control with an intracortical neural interface system by humans with tetraplegia [45]	2011	USA
Control of a visual keyboard using an electrocorticographic brain-computer interface [44]	2011	USA
A wireless brain-machine interface for real-time speech synthesis [46]	2009	USA
Robust, long-term control of an electrocorticographic brain-computer interface with fixed parameters [47]	2009	USA
Electrocorticographically controlled brain-computer interfaces using motor and sensory imagery in patients with temporary subdural electrode implants. Report of four cases [48]	2007	USA
Electrocorticography-based brain computer interface—the Seattle experience [49]	2006	USA

3.2. Intracortical Implants

A total of 15 studies examined the effects of the implantation of intracortical BCIs into patients [10,11,13,21,25,28,30,32,34–36,38,40,42,45,46], and all electrodes used were supplied by BlackRock Neurotech (Table 2). Notably, none had functional movement in the upper and lower limbs. There were 29 separate cases on the patients involved. In total, 10 looked at patients suffering from ALS [11,21,34–36,38,45], 6 assessed patients with brainstem stroke [35,38,40,42,45,46], and 13 included patients with spinal cord injury [10,13,25,28,30,32,34,36].

Patients with spinal cord injuries had C4–C6 injuries (Table 2) that left them with poor control of their extremities. The monitoring of neural instability prompting recalibration was demonstrated, which can make monitoring patients more efficient [10]. Additionally, in two studies, the supramarginal gyrus (SMG) was also shown as an anatomical target, suggesting the SMG not only holds an internalised representation of vocalised and internal speech, but the neural signals can also be used for speech BMIs [13,25]. Wireless implantation that allowed patients with severe motor impairment to live in the community was demonstrated [30].

When controlling a cursor on the screen to select targets, it is possible to achieve up to approximately 24 characters per minute by optimising user interface. Simply adapting a keyboard that has closer targets such as the opti-II keyboard significantly increases the speed of selection [36]. This is particularly relevant as the surveying of ALS patients suggests that 72% would be satisfied with a speed of 15–19 correct characters/min [50]. The motor cortex can be targeted for the movement of a cursor through motor imagery, with users achieving a minimum syllable recognition accuracy of 54.7% and similarly a minimum word decoding accuracy of 61.5%, with variations among patients perhaps suggestive of the need to optimise other factors that can affect performance. Further research is required to elucidate these results [32].

Additionally, the SMG has been shown to be an important target for decoding words, with chronic implantation achieving up to 79% average decoding accuracy, and is found to be a common anatomical landmark for internal and vocalised speech, as well as grasp motor imagery, suggesting dual purposes [25].

Table 2. Details on intracortical implants for spinal cord injury patients.

Age and Gender	Injury	Number of Electrodes and Anatomical Placement	Electrode Details	Behaviour Task	Outcome
37M [10] 65M [10]	C4 AIS-B spinal cord injury (SCI) C4 AIS-C SCI	1 × 96 channel in hand/arm knob of dominant (left) precentral gyrus	Not reported	Attempt hand/finger movement to move cursor	The novel decoder recalibration method quantifies and monitors instability in neural recording, suggesting when recalibration should take place.
33M [13] 39M [13]	C5 spinal cord injury C6 spinal cord injury	1 × 96 in left SMG 1 × 96 in left ventral premotor cortex 2 × 48 in left hand/arm of S1 1 × 64 in left SMG, 1 × 64 in left ventral premotor cortex, 1 × 64 in primary motor cortex, 2 × 64 in left S1	Platinum-tipped or sputtered iridium oxide film (SIROF)-tipped	Internally and externally vocalise words	The offline accuracy of recording from the SMG was 24% and 55% for each patient. This increased with an online internal speech task as users achieved 25% and 79% decoding accuracy. This suggests significant neural representation in internal and vocalised speech at the SMG. Additionally, activity in the somatosensory cortex (S1) was present during vocalised but not internalised speech, suggesting that no articulatory movement of the vocal tract occurred during internal speech.
Age not reported [25]	C5 cervical spinal cord injury	1 × 96 in SMG, 1 × 96 in PMv, 2 × 48 in S1	Iridium oxide	Motor imagery of grasps meaning he imagined making the hand shapes without actually moving	The patient, who was unable to physically move his hands due to tetraplegia, was asked to perform motor imagery of the grasps. The results showed that individual grasps could be decoded from the neural activity in all three brain regions, indicating their potential as target sites for grasp BMIs. They found that the SMG could also decode spoken grasp names, suggesting its potential role in speech BMIs. This contrasted with PMv and S1, which did not have a significant classification of speech for colours or grasp names.

Table 2. *Cont.*

Age and Gender	Injury	Number of Electrodes and Anatomical Placement	Electrode Details	Behaviour Task	Outcome
Age not reported [28]	C5 motor/C6 sensory ASIA B spinal cord injury	2 × 88 in hand and arm areas of motor cortex	Not reported	Motor imagery using arm to move cursor and grasp to click	This study investigated the use of transient neural responses at the onset and offset of an attempted hand grasp to provide more generalizable click control for intracortical brain–computer interfaces. The researchers developed a novel, transient-based click decoder and compared its performance to the standard sustained click decoder. This research provides evidence that a transient-based approach to click decoding can significantly improve iBCI control by enabling both discrete and sustained click functionality.
Age not reported [28]	C6 ASIA B spinal cord injury	2 × 96 implanted in hand area of motor cortex	Not reported		
63M [30]	C4 AIS-C spinal cord injury	2 × 96 implanted in left (dominant) precentral gyrus	Platinum tips	Point and click of commercial apps using cursor at home	The study found that the wireless system could effectively record and decode neural signals, allowing participants to control a computer cursor and a tablet computer. The performance of the wireless system was comparable to that of the wired system in terms of accuracy and speed. The successful implementation of the wireless system in a home setting marks a significant step towards developing more practical and user-friendly assistive technologies for people with severe motor impairments.
35M [30]	C4 AIS-A SCI		Platinum tips		
64M [32]	C4 AIS-C SCI	2 × 96 implanted in dorsal hand knob area of left (dominant) motor cortex	1.5 mm electrode	Patient attempted speech and orofacial movement when prompted	The study shows the hand knob motor area of the motor cortex to also be responsible for speech production. Patient 1 had an accuracy of syllables of 84.6% and word decoding of 83.5%. Patient 2 had an accuracy of syllables of 54.7% and 61.5% of word decoding.
56M [32]	C4 AIS-A SCI		1.5 mm electrode		

Table 2. *Cont.*

Age and Gender	Injury	Number of Electrodes and Anatomical Placement	Electrode Details	Behaviour Task	Outcome
63M [34]	C4 ASIA-C	1 × 96 implanted in hand and arm area of dominant (left) motor cortex	1 mm electrode	Motor imagery using hand/arm flexion to control cursor	The study looked at three patients including two ALS and one spinal cord injury patient using a point and click device on a commercial tablet. Patients were able to select 8.3–25.3 words per minute but also used other mediums such as email, chat, browsing the web, and accessing weather, news, music, and videos.
63M [36]	C4 ASIA-C	2 × 96 implanted into upper extremity area of dominant (left) motor cortex	1.5 mm intracortical silicon microelectrode	Move cursor on screen to type	When free typing, one patient was able to achieve 24.4 ± 3.3 characters per minute. Two patients using Opti-II keyboard performed quicker than when using a qwerty keyboard. One patient performed quicker using an abcdef keyborard than when using opti-II, but the patient had minimal typing experience beforehand.

Intracortical implants were also used for patients suffering from ALS (Table 3). The Revised Amyotrophic Lateral Sclerosis Functional Rating Scale (ALSFRS-R) score ranged from 6 to 23 [11,34–36]. The ALSFR scale demonstrates the severity of ALS on a scale of 0–40, with a higher scale demonstrating greater retained function. Two cases looked at patients attempting to speak [11,21], whilst seven [34–36,38,45] looked at patients attempting to move a cursor. Six cases involved the implantation of a 96-channel electrode [35,36,38,42,45], one study implanted a 4 × 64 channel electrode implant [11], and one study implanted 2 × 96 electrodes [34]. Earlier studies examined the ability of patients with ALS to communicate by controlling a cursor using an implanted BCI. One study showed patients achieving a word selection of 8.3–25.3 words per min and an ability to communicate using common digital solutions such as email, internet browsing, etc. [34]. In another study, patients achieved 6.88 correct characters/min but demonstrated no need for recalibration over 138 days [35]. Auto-calibration being comparable to a standard decoder is also demonstrated in two more patients in a separate study [38]. The importance of keyboard selection is also demonstrated as patients were able to achieve an increase in speed of up to 1.3× when using a Opti-II keyboard compared to a QWERTY keyboard [36]. However, this has proven to be slow and requires considerable effort. Later studies that attempted to decode words proved to have a much greater accuracy and speed. In one study, patients achieved an accuracy of 97.5% using a 125,000 word vocabulary [11]. Another study showed a patient being able to communicate at a rate of 62 words per minute, which is significantly higher than the results obtained with cursor control [21].

Patients with brainstem strokes also have a similar functional basis to those with ALS and spinal cord injuries. Most of these studies looked at motor imagery where patients were asked to move a cursor on a screen (Table 4). The focus of the implantation was in the precentral gyrus [35,40,42,45,46], with the aim of taking advantage of the neural recordings that occurred in the arm/hand area of the motor cortex. While high accuracy can be achieved, low speed hampers the performance. Self-calibration can be used to avoid the need for constant calibration, and results comparable to a standard decoder can be achieved [38]. One study demonstrated the potential of patients choosing approximately 3 correct characters/min to communicate [35], whilst another had rates of 2.7–8.6 correct selections/min but also demonstrated successful results 1000 days after implantation [42,45]. The importance of choosing a correct keyboard design was again demonstrated with radial keyboards outperforming the QWERTY keyboard [40].

Table 3. Details on intracortical implants for ALS patients.

Age and Gender	Extent of ALS	Number of Electrodes Anatomical Placement	Electrode Details	Behaviour Task	Outcome
45M [11]	Tetraparesis + severe dyarthria ALS functional rating scale revised (ALSFRS-R) score is 23	256 electrodes in left precentral gyrus—patient was confirmed to be left hemisphere language-dominant by fMRI	4 microelectrodes with each measuring 3.2 × 3.2 mm in size and electrode depth 1.5 mm	Attempt to speak	The BCI achieved an accuracy of 99.6% using a 50-word vocabulary. With training, the accuracy was 97.5% using a 125,000-word vocabulary. Arrays in the ventral premotor cortex and middle precentral gyrus contributed most to decoding accuracy.
51F [34]	ALSFRS-R score is 14—retained speech and dexterous movement of wrist and some fingers	96-channel electrodes in hand area of dominant (left) motor cortex	1 mm electrode length, 4 × 4 mm	Motor imagery using hand/arm flexion to control cursor	The study looked at three patients using a point and click device on a commercial tablet. Patients were able to select 8.3–25.3 words per minute but also used other mediums such as email, chat, browsing the web, and accessing weather, news, music, and videos.
51M [34]	ALSFRS-R score is 6—retained speech but minimal movement in hands/fingers	2 × 96 electrodes in hand area of dominant (left) motor cortex	1.5 mm electrode length	Motor imagery using hand/arm flexion to control cursor	
Age not reported [35]	ALSFRS-R score is 16—had tracheostomy and on-demand ventilation. She could speak but had limited hand mobility	96 channel electrode into arm area of dominant precentral gyrus	Not reported	Move cursor on screen	The study looked at intracortical local field potentials where the patient averaged one word per minute without the need for recalibration and sustained performance over several months. The study lasted for 138 days. Spelling rates of 6.88 correct characters/minute allowed the patient to also type messages and write emails.
51F [36]	ALSFRS-R score is 16—retained dexterous movement of hand and wrist	96 channel electrode into hand area of dominant (left) motor cortex	1.0 mm silicon electrode	Move cursor on screen to type	When free typing, the patient was able to achieve 24.4 ± 3.3 characters per minute using an Opti-II keyboard. This was 1.3 times quicker than when using a QWERTY keyboard.
54M [36]	ALSFRS-R score is 17—very limited movement in fingers	96 channel electrode implanted into hand area of dominant (left) motor cortex	1.5 mm silicon electrode	Move cursor on screen to type	The patient performed quicker using an ABCDEF keyboard than when using a QWERTY keyboard. However, the patient also had limited typing experience beforehand.
51F [38]	Not reported	96 channel electrode implanted into hand/arm knob area of dominant motor cortex	1.0 mm electrodes	Selecting character on screen	The auto-calibration of the decoder using a retrospective decoder produced comparable accuracy (12 characters correct per minute) as a standard decoder (11.4 correct characters/minute). Even with longer trials involving self-typing sessions, i.e., 1–2+ h, typing rates remained high.
58M [38]	Not reported		1.5 mm electrode		
37M [45]	Paralysis	96 channel electrode implanted into arm area of dominant motor cortex	Not reported	Move cursor by imaging being able to control the cursor and click by imaging right hand opening	In total, 52.6% of targets were selected correctly but failed only due to time-out. The false-click average was one per trial.
67F [21]	Patient has bulbar onset ALS. Whilst she retains some limited orofacial movement and can vocalise, she has an inability to produce intelligible speech	2 × 64 channel electrode implanted ventral premotor cortex (area 6v) and 2 × 64 channel electrodes in area 44	3.2 mm arrays	Attempt at speech	The patient was able to communicate at a rate of 62 words per minute, which was significantly higher than previous approaches. She had a 23.8% error rate on a vocabulary consisting of 125,000 words.

Table 4. Details on intracortical implants for brainstem stroke patients.

Age and Gender	Stroke Pathology	Number of Electrodes Anatomical Placement	Electrode Details	Behaviour Task	Outcome
Age not reported [35]	Brainstem stroke leading to locked-in syndrome	96-channel electrode into arm area of dominant precentral gyrus	Not reported	Moving cursor on screen	The study looked at intracortical local field potentials where the patient averaged one word per minute without the need for recalibration, and sustained performance over several months. Study lasted for 76 days. Spelling rates of 3.07 correct characters/minute allowed patient to also type messages and write emails.
57F [38]	Not reported		1.5 mm electrode tips	Selecting character on screen	The auto-calibration of the decoder using a retrospective decoder produced comparable accuracy (12 characters correct per minute) as a standard decoder (11.4 correct characters/minute).
66M [38]	Not reported		1.5 mm electrode tips		
58F [40]	Bilateral pontine infarction	96-channel implanted in the arm/hand area of her motor cortex	Not reported	Moving cursor on screen by attempting to move dominant hand at wrist	Using a radial keyboard led to an improvement of 65% in correct characters selected per minute and outperformed the QWERTY keyboard in all tasks. The patient was also able to use the keyboard to enter google chat and communicate at a rate of 8.1 correct characters per minute
56F [42]	Brainstem stroke leading to anarthria and tetraplegia	96-channel implanted in arm area of motor cortex	Not reported	Moving cursor on screen by attempting to move dominant right hand and right hand grasp to select	After 1000 days post implantation, the BCI was still working well. The patient was able to successfully select 2.7–8.6 correct selections/minute on a screen at a success rate of 91.9–94.9% over 5 days.
26M [46]	Brainstem stroke leading to locked-in syndrome	Neurotrophic electrode implanted into precentral gyrus	Single 3-wire electrode	Attempted speech patterns were wirelessly transmitted and converted in real time using a Kalman filter-decoder	The participant significantly improved their performance of a vowel production task over a 1.5 h period involving 34 or fewer vowels, increasing the average accuracy from 45% to 70%.
55F [45]	Brainstem stroke leading to tetraplegia	96-channel electrode implanted into arm area of dominant motor cortex	Not reported	Moving cursor by imaging being able to control the cursor and click by imaging right hand closing	In total, 97.4% of the targets were selected correctly but failed only due to time-out. The false-click average was 0.74 per trial. It took the patient 7.2 ± 3.8 s seconds to move the cursor over a distance of 12 cm.

3.3. ECoG-Based Studies

ECoG arrays were initially used in patients with epilepsy, and surgeons placed them according to patient needs as oppose to research purposes. However, the discoveries from these have led to significant improvements in our understanding of how speech is modulated in the brain [19,22,24,47,49]. Additionally, the studies also demonstrated that patients were able to control virtual keyboards even with ECoG devices outside of the language centre [51]. Anatomical regions including the ventral sensorimotor cortex (vSMC), superior temporal gyrus (STG) and inferior frontal gyrus (IFG) were demonstrated to be areas involved in language production when patients only mime the sounds [33]. Gesture prediction was higher than phoneme prediction overall, but anatomically, gesture prediction was substantially more accurate in the posterior areas of the cortex (corresponding largely to the primary sensorimotor and part of premotor cortices), whilst in more anterior areas, the performances for both gesture and phoneme prediction were more similar [39].

ECoG-based BCIs were also implanted in patients with ALS and stroke (Table 5). In patients with ALS, subdural electrodes were places over the sensorimotor cortex [14,16,18] and prefrontal cortex [16]. On the other hand, a pontine stroke patient had a high-density (hdECoG) array covering the left precentral gyrus, postcentral gyrus, posterior middle frontal gyrus, and posterior inferior frontal gyrus [29], while another pontine infarct patient had subdural electrodes covering the posterior aspect of the middle frontal gyrus, precentral gyrus, and anterior aspect of the postcentral gyrus, as well as the dorsal posterior aspect of the inferior frontal gyrus [23], and the final patient with a bilateral pontine stroke had implantation in the region of the dorsal posterior aspect of the inferior frontal gyrus, posterior aspect of the middle frontal gyrus, precentral gyrus, and anterior aspect of the postcentral gyrus [12]. In contrast to intracortical implants, ECoG arrays covered larger areas of the brain, although a study suggested the control of a cursor through a single subdural electrode strip with four electrodes measuring 4 mm each [41]. ECoG arrays are also able to convert attempted speech production directly into words spelled at a rate of 29.4 characters/min and a character error rate of 6.13% [23], whilst another study demonstrated the successful decoding of bilingual speech for both English and Spanish phrases [12], suggesting that the speech BCI can be used for languages other than English. The impact of recurrent neural networks to convert attempted speech into acoustic speech is demonstrated [14].

Furthermore, one study demonstrated the significance of the dorsolateral prefrontal cortex (dlPFC) as an anatomical target for BCIs for cursor control [43]. The potential benefits of using dlPFC in BCIs include providing an alternative target in cases where surgeons are unable to utilise the sensorimotor signals. This approach offers an alternative communication pathway for individuals with LIS who may have difficulty modulating sensorimotor activity due to their neurological conditions. Additionally, both participants reported finding dlPFC-based BCI control less mentally taxing than sensorimotor-based control.

Using predictive algorithms also helped with speed as spelling initially took 52 s per letter, but the time required dropped to 33 s per letter when word prediction was used. Crucially, the system could be used when the existing mode of communication failed as seen whenever she went outside, where lighting conditions made eye tracking impossible. The patient also expressed greater satisfaction with the BCI than eye-tracking system [37].

Table 5. ECoG implantation in patients to aid communication.

Age and Gender	Pathology	Number of Electrodes Anatomical Placement	Behaviour Task	Outcome
60M [14]	ALS: ALSFRS-R score of 26: Patient had primarily disability of bulbar and upper extremity muscle, resulting in mostly unintelligible speech	Two 8 × 8 subdural electrodes covering ventral sensorimotor cortex and representative dorsal laryngeal area using platinum–iridium disc electrodes covering 36.6 mm × 33.1 mm	Patient was tasked with reading aloud words in a closed vocabulary of 6 words	Using a recurrent neural network, the BCI was able to produce acoustic speech that included the characteristics and natural pacing of the patient's speech. Native English speakers could interpret the attempted words with 80% accuracy from the synthesised speech.
35F [48]	Epilepsy with right anterior temporal lobe lesion	Subdural in right temporal lobe	Motor imagery to move cursor on screen	Cursor control can be achieved with minimal training. In this study, participants trained for 45 min in a day for a total of 2–7 days.
43M [48]	Epilepsy with left temporal lobe tumour	Subdural in left temporal lobe		
18F [48]	Epilepsy with left temporal lobe mass	Left perisylvian region		
60F [48]	Medically intractable facial pain	Right primary motor cortex		
58F [16]	ALS: ALSFRS-R score of 1	2 electrode strips over the dorsolateral prefrontal cortex and 2 over the sensorimotor cortex	Control of a cursor on a monitor and clicking	This was an update on a previous study where the patient had used the BCI to communicate with family and caregivers. This included calling for medication or requesting airway suction. After approximately 6 years of use, the signals' quality started to decrease, coinciding with atrophy in frontal and parietal brain volume, leading to increased distance between strips (that were attached to the skull) and cortex.
61M [18]	ALS patient with bulbar dysfunction, leading to severe progressive dysarthria and dyspnoea	2 × 64 channel subdural with each strip covering a surface area of 36.66 mm × 33.1 mm over the ventral sensorimotor cortex	Patient read single text commands aloud or mimed them as they appeared on a computer monitor	Speech was accurately decoded with a median accuracy of 90.59% over a 3 month period without the need for recalibration. No adverse effects were also observed from implantation throughout the 3-month period.

Table 5. *Cont.*

Age and Gender	Pathology	Number of Electrodes Anatomical Placement	Behaviour Task	Outcome
36M [12]	Bilateral pontine stroke: patient was left with severe spastic quadriparesis and anarthria	hdECoG array implanted subdurally using a total of 128 electrodes and was centred to sample from dorsal posterior aspect of inferior frontal gyrus, posterior aspect of middle frontal gyrus, precentral gyrus, and anterior aspect of postcentral gyrus	Patient attempted to speak words throughout the tasks	The decoding of bilingual speech led to a median word error rate of 25.0% across online testing blocks for both English and Spanish phrases, demonstrating the system's ability to decode intended speech in both languages. The system could freely decode the intended language with a median accuracy of 87.5% based on neural features and the differential linguistic context built throughout a phrase. A comparison between the speed of this BCI and the participant's previous communication method, an augmentative and alternative communication (AAC) interface that used residual head movements to spell words, was also made. The BCI achieved a median speed of 21 words per minute, which was considerably faster than the participant's AAC rate of 3 words per minute
47F [20]	Pontine infarction with left vertebral artery dissection and basilar artery occlusion—patient is unable to articulate intelligible words	hdECoG array with 253 electrodes implanted to cover regions associated with speech and language including left middle aspect of the superior and middle temporal gyri, the precentral gyrus and the postcentral gyrus	Activation of neurons was recorded with attempts to silently voice words from 249 randomly selected words by moving orofacial muscles including that of the tongue, lips, and jaw.	The study involved multiple stages of recording signals for word production. The system decodes the neural signals and displays the intended words as text on a screen. Speech Audio: The system synthesises audible speech from the participant's brain activity. Facial Avatar Animation: The system animates a virtual avatar to accompany the synthesised speech, creating a more embodied communication experience. The avatar can display both speech-related and non-speech facial gestures, including emotional expressions.

Table 5. *Cont.*

Age and Gender	Pathology	Number of Electrodes Anatomical Placement	Behaviour Task	Outcome
36M [23]	Extensive pontine infarct leading to severe spastic quadriparesis and anarthria	hdECoG with 128 electrodes covering the left hemisphere associated with speech production. This includes the posterior aspect of the middle frontal gyrus, the precentral gyrus, and the anterior aspect of the postcentral gyrus, as well as the dorsal posterior aspect of the inferior frontal gyrus.	Patient attempted to start speaking	The primary goal was to assess if the participant could use silent attempts to speak to control the BCI and spell out intended messages from a 1152-word vocabulary. The system achieved a median character error rate of 6.13% and a median word error rate of 10.53% during the copy-typing task. The median spelling rate was 29.4 characters per minute and 6.9 words per minute, exceeding the participant's typing speed with his existing assistive device. Silent Control: This study is the first to demonstrate successful sentence decoding from silent speech attempts, paving the way for communication restoration in individuals with complete vocal tract paralysis.
36M [29]	Pontine stroke associated with dissection of right vertebral artery	128 electrodes placed in subdural space over left sensorimotor cortex including left precentral gyrus, postcentral gyrus, posterior middle frontal gyrus, and posterior inferior frontal gyrus	Attempted speech production	The BCI system successfully decoded full sentences from the participant's cortical activity in real time. The median rate of decoding was 15.2 words per minute, with a median word error rate of 25.6%.
58F [43]	ALS patient with ALSFRS-R score of 2	Subdural placement in left prefrontal cortex and left sensorimotor cortex	Cursor movement	The study demonstrated the use of the dorsolateral prefrontal cortex (dlPFC) as an anatomical target to control a cursor in a one-dimensional BCI task. This task involved moving a cursor up or down by either performing serial subtraction or resting.
39F [43]	Pontine stroke leading to tetraplegia			

Table 5. *Cont.*

Age and Gender	Pathology	Number of Electrodes Anatomical Placement	Behaviour Task	Outcome
58F [37]	ALS patient with ALSFRS-R score of 2	Subdural electrodes placed over the hand region of the left motor cortex, and left prefrontal region	Cursor movement	The study looked at communication for an ALS patient with LIS. The patient used the BCI for 262 days. The patient was able to achieve an accuracy of 89 $\pm$ 6% of the time, with the subjective mental effort required decreasing from an initial 5 to 2.8 out of 5.
36F, 49M, 45F, 48F [31]	Epilepsy	Subdural positioned strip consisting of 64 (8 $\times$ 8) electrodes positioned on left lateral surface	Patients controlled a cursor by expressing a series of phonemes	Regions coding for phonemes included Wernicke's area (BA 40), the auditory cortex (BA 42 and BA 22), premotor cortex (BA 6), and sensorimotor cortex (BA 3). All patients achieved accuracy greater than 69% after 4 to 15 min of closed-loop control experiments when deciphering phonemes.

3.4. SEEG-Based Studies

sEEG has also been utilised as a tool in this domain. A particular advantage of this method is that sEEG devices have already been successfully implanted in patients for multiple years, as seen in the treatment of Parkinson's disease [52].

The electrode size is approximately akin to that of surface EEG devices, although there may be a limit to the number of electrodes used to record signals for desired functional outcomes [15,17,26]. One study found a logarithmic relationship between the number of neurons that the electrodes recorded from and decoding accuracy. This means that increasing the number of neurons improved the accuracy, but the gains were greater with smaller neuron counts. The finding suggests that there is a point of diminishing returns when the number of recorded neurons for decoding is increased. The left Vim exhibited involvement in all three aspects of speech: production, perception, and imagery. While speech production decoding yielded the highest accuracies, likely because of the targeting of motor areas within the left Vim, the high accuracies for perception and imagery (96% and 80%, respectively) suggest that the left Vim plays a role beyond motor control in speech processing. The study discovered that vowels 'e' and 'u' were more frequently confused during decoding than other vowels, suggesting these vowels might share similar neuronal representations in the left Vim. This finding could inform future research on vowel encoding and decoding in the thalamus and contribute to refining decoding algorithms [15]. Additionally, a BCI speller using only three electrodes placed over the middle temporal visual area was able to achieve a speed of 12 characters/min, comparable to other BCIs controlling cursors [24]. For deep brain stimulation electrodes implanted in the subthalamic nucleus, it may also be possible to decode speech information from the electrical activity of single neurons in the subthalamic nucleus of patients with Parkinson's disease. One study showed the accurate decoding of vowels during speech production (100% accuracy), speech perception (96% accuracy) and speech imagery (88% accuracy). Neuronal activity could therefore accurately predict vowel sounds that participants produced, perceived or imagined [26]. Other targets of speech decoding include the posterior hippocampal region [44]. In this study, the authors demonstrated the synthesised output corresponded in real time with utterance timings, suggesting reliable audible speech generation. However, reconstructed audio was not intelligible [27], seemingly because of using simple decoding methods. However, the study used simple decoding methods. Future studies that incorporate the use of deep learning-integrated decoding methods could provide clearer audio output. Nonetheless, this study is important in suggesting that sEEG targeting the hippocampal region can be utilised for speech production and can provide a platform on which future studies can build upon.

4. Discussion

This review focused on intracortical BCIs used for communication. Whilst earlier studies demonstrated the use of cursor control to allow the selection of characters on a screen (Figure 2), later studies have gone a step further and allowed direct speech-to-text and speech-to-audio conversion (Figure 3). However, whilst these allow users to communicate at a rate of approximately 62 words/min [21], it still falls short of natural speech production which averages 120–150 words/min. For patients, this potentially means quicker and more seamless communication, although to achieve this, the BCI package must also incorporate modern computing methods such as the use of deep neural networks and engineering solutions that allow higher-fidelity electrodes to facilitate better signal pick-up [20].

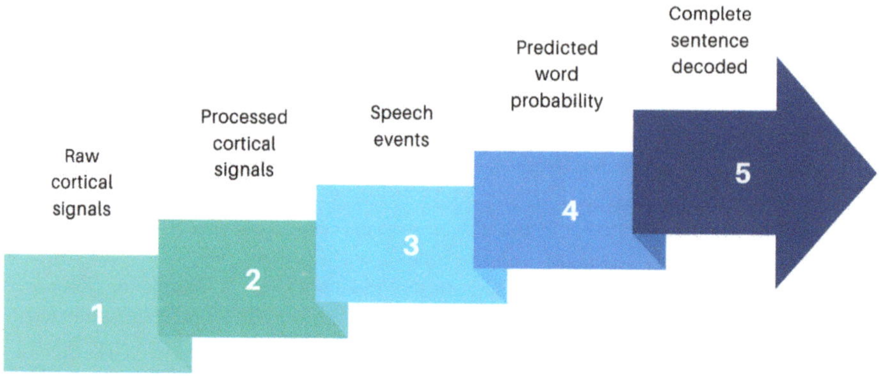

Figure 3. Signal processing sequences for sentence decoding: adapted from Moses and colleagues [29]. Sequential analysis from collection of raw cortical data to output of complete sentences. Raw broadband cortical signals are initially picked up by electrodes placed over the speech sensorimotor cortex. Neural signals are processed to remove noise and form meaningful processed cortical signals. Computation algorithms can then convert these processed signals into speech events by detecting speech patterns to form words. Using deep neural networks improves the success probability, and predicted words sequenced together alongside probabilistic modelling packages can allow complete sentence decoding. Sentence structures can be fed into output devices such as avatars or speech articulators to allow meaningful communication in a more natural manner.

Non-invasive technologies such as EEG, fMRI, and magnetoencephalography (MEG) do not require surgical implantation. fMRI has high spatial specificity, allowing anatomical localisation, but its low temporal resolution means that tracking neural changes at the millisecond level is difficult because of the lag in cerebral blood flow, and it also currently requires access to an MRI scanner [53]. However, MEG and EEG suffer from low spatial specificity although they have high temporal resolution [54,55]. From a practical perspective, EEG offers portability and can therefore be translated to patients in the real world. However, difficulty associated with diminishing noise means there is likely going to be a limit to scaling the accurate decoding of large vocabularies and longer speech segments. As such, invasive BCIs offer an attractive solution to overcome these deficiencies from non-invasive devices (Figure 4).

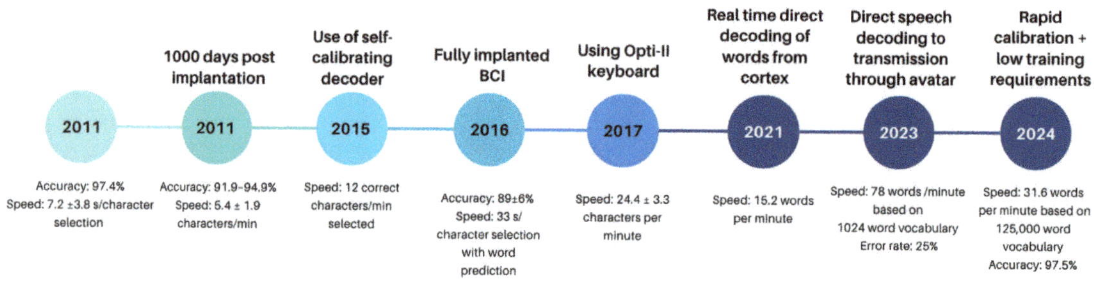

Figure 4. Timeline showing major advances in the field of invasive BCIs for communication. There has been a big leap forward in the rate of speech production due to direct cortex to speech production as opposed to the earlier studies that relied on cursor control. There remains heterogeneity in variables that authors choose to publish, which makes it difficult to compare outcomes.

Invasive BCIs, which are separated into ECoG, intracortical, and sEEG, offer distinct advantages and disadvantages, and an ad hoc approach depending on patient needs may be beneficial. ECoG electrodes can offer high spatial resolution, typically at the millimetre scale. Furthermore, they allow the possibility of a large area to be covered, as the number of electrodes can often be tailored from dozens to hundreds of electrodes. On the other hand, sEEG typically provides sparser coverage but can record from deeper structures including limbic structures. Additionally, ECoG is often implanted to cover the unilateral recording of a cerebral hemisphere, whilst sEEG can be implanted bilaterally [56,57].

Recording from the arm/hand area of the motor cortex during controlling a cursor for communication has been well demonstrated, although the greatest disadvantage is slower speed. To improve speed, research has shifted towards the direct interpretation of speech from cortical recordings, and indeed, high-performance speech decoding is possible from recordings in the anterior precentral gyrus [11,21,32].

Anatomically, because there are multiple regions of the brain that are involved in speech production, there may exist multiple targets for implantation, although further research is required to elucidate the extent to which each region can provide speech rehabilitation. Input to the vSMC and middle precentral gyrus (midPrCG) is received from the superior temporal gyrus and supramarginal gyrus. Somatotopically arranged neural populations sit along the vSMC and middle precentral gyrus, forming the corticobulbar system [58,59]. They play an important role in controlling vocal tract articulators including the tongue, jaw, lips, and larynx, which work in a coordinated manner to produce speech driven by expired air. Dorsally located is the region that controls hand movement [60,61], although targeting this region is more appropriate for the on-screen control of cursors. Given the large number of regions that are involved in speech production, targeting the intact regions may be a viable method for speech decoding. Placing an ECoG array therefore provides an advantage given the large coverage that is possible including the vSMC, superior temporal gyrus, and midPrCG with a single array.

Studies have also demonstrated the at-home use of these device [30]. Along with decoders that can auto-calibrate [38], it allows patients to live a more normal life in an environment in which they are more comfortable. As such, translation to a real-life clinical scenario is more likely with devices that are unrestrictive in terms of location.

Additionally, it is evident that accurate decoding using modern solutions including artificial intelligence will substantially improve BCI clinical outcomes [38]. In addition, studies should focus on improving the user experience, which includes the interface and ease with which patients can interact with the device. This will likely lead to significant improvements in speed and accuracy [36].

An important consideration that should be acknowledged is the surgical risks that are also associated with the implantation of invasive BCI devices (Table 6). Whilst surgical implantation techniques will likely be optimised to reduce invasiveness and minimise intra-operative risks to patients, current methods of implantation involve a craniotomy approach to expose large areas of cortical tissue. Surgical risks include the risk of infection, bleeding, and damage to eloquent areas. This can also have an impact on the devices themselves as intracortical implants such as microelectrodes can elicit inflammatory responses, leading to scarring and the loss of neurons [62,63].

Table 6. Left hand column lists major surgical considerations for invasive BCIs. Right hand column lists the major ethical categories for invasive BCIs.

Surgical Considerations	Ethical Considerations
Infection Bleeding Iatrogenic damage Inflammation Anaesthetic complications Postoperative pain Lengthy rehabilitation	Legal justice: Regulatory agencies control the introduction of neurotechnologies into trials and clinical practice. Once on the market, continuous safety monitoring as well as ethical issues arising on cases of malpractice, hacking, and the mis-use of data will remain a subject of concern. Distributive justice: Neurotechnologies that are used for enhancement purposes may create a societal divide where select individuals are able to achieve improved characteristics such as strength, cognition, or connection to external devices. Autonomy: The stimulation of cortical tissue can lead to changes in thought patterns, and as such, there is plausibility for altered decision making under the influence of neurotechnologies.

The long-term efficacy of BCIs is a topic of research. Inflammation after implantation likely will contribute to the chronic stability of recordings, but this could also be dependent on the implantation technique such as the disruption of microvasculature as the device is implanted. With ECoG devices, impedance will likely stabilise after several months [64–66]. Intracortical devices also have additional unique challenges. Surgical implantation is of greater significance as factors such as the size, material, and shape of electrodes, insertion speed, and roughness of the implantable device can lead to an acute inflammatory response [67–69]. Thus, immediately after insertion, neurons directly in contact can be killed, which can significantly reduce the neuron population. Subsequent glial response can further propagate the inflammatory response. Additionally, as the device is often tethered, electrodes are fixed whilst the brain can move independently, causing further damage to the brain through these micromotions. Over time, a glial scar with a size of ~100 μm can form, which creates a further barrier between the electrode and the brain, increasing the space between neurons and electrodes [70–72]. This can lead to worsening signal quality, through neural displacement, electrical insulation, and the modulation of neighbouring neurons. During this phase, there is typically an increase in electrical impedance, although this stabilises over the following months. However, despite the decline in signal quality, the impact on users' functional performance may not be linear, as participants are able to maintain high BCI performance many months/years after insertion [66].

However, patient pathology may also contribute to worsening signal quality. This is particularly evident in cases where the brain will atrophy such as in ALS. If the electrodes are fixed to the skull, the sensors can migrate from the region of interest if the brain atrophies as with ALS, thereby limiting the functional use of the BCI [16]. Therefore, the clinical translation of devices will benefit from wireless implantation devices.

Lastly, the studies lack homogeneity when discussing different tasks performed by a user which makes comparisons difficult. The choice of behavioural tasks on brain performance is an important consideration in neurotechnology research because the choice of task can have a large impact on decoding accuracy and speed and overall system reliability, which greatly affects patient performance. More complex tasks will also require greater cognitive effort. Additionally, the nature of the task is also important. Using motor imagery whereby users mentally rehearse movement to invoke event-related desynchronization (ERD) and synchronisation (ERS) patterns in the sensorimotor cortex involves different levels of training and mental effort compared to speech decoding, but a comparison between these tasks is difficult without standardised behavioural task protocols. This includes using metrics such as session duration, the number of trials, rest intervals, feedback mechanisms, and control conditions to account for spontaneous neural activity fluctuations. Performance metrics should also be standardised, which not only includes objective data such as characters/min and speed but also user fatigue and cognitive load. Therefore, the development of consensus guidelines for the reporting of BCI performance is required and would greatly enhance comparability and reproducibility across studies.

5. Ethics

As the field of BCIs evolves, a range of ethical issues has to be addressed (Table 6). Whilst this is not the focus of this review, we include it here as a point of discussion to raise awareness. Implantable BCIs pose further concerns in comparison to non-invasive technologies as the surgical risks must also be considered. Invasive BCIs have the potential to enhance the ability of users [73]. Whilst the studies performed thus far have been on patients suffering from a neurological deficit, it is possible to adapt the studies for healthy participants to facilitate connection with external devices. This can lead to, for instance, the ability to control a robotic arm or computer screen through thought. Justifying surgical risks for such procedures can be considered adjacent to cosmetic procedures that may not be life-saving but performed if patients desire it. However, the ability to record and stimulate the nervous system has wider implications including societal risks.

Enhancing individuals beyond their natural limitations can be seen by some as going against limitations set naturally. If such technology was only accessibly to select few due to limited access or high costs, it can create a divide in society where individuals who have neuroenhancement may be seen as superior or be able to have a wider repertoire of functions available to them [8]. This ties in with the concept of distributive justice. From a utilitarian perspective, if only select individuals have access to technologies that allow them the ability to enhance themselves, the large divide in society can be more detrimental than the potential positive that it can bring. This can be seen, for example, with enhancement drugs such as stimulants that allow students to gain an advantage over their peers [74].

Furthermore, as BCIs have the ability to collect neuro-data, it can provide a rich source of data for commercial uses, such as consumer targeting. Additionally, neural signals are closely aligned with an individual's identity, and as such, the use of these data can infringe upon patient confidentiality [8,75].

Finally, as BCIs can be connected with other digital devices, it opens up the possibility of hacking and infringing upon user autonomy. This is already a concern with other implantable devices such as insulin pumps and pacemakers [76,77]. Because the brain is such a complex organ, hacking and accessing neuro-data as well as stimulating nervous tissue can have severe and unpredictable consequences.

It is therefore imperative that regulation of BCIs is given priority and continuously updated as our understanding of neuroscience improves and neurotechnology evolves.

6. Conclusions

BCIs provide a significant therapeutic option for patients who otherwise have limited rehabilitation recovery. However, over the last decade, the pace of this field has been rapid and has shifted from cursor control to the decoding of speech directly from the brain in a bid to improve the speed of communication. The ability to facilitate communication in a neurologically impaired patient can significantly improve their quality of life. However, significant resources are required to achieve greater results. Interpreting high-quality signals and decoding them to speech requires innovative solutions such as the incorporation of AI to reduce noise and improve language interpretation, as well as optimising the user interface to allow patients to interact better with the software in a more natural manner. However, costly innovations may run the risk of secluding patients who cannot access this technology, which can create a societal divide. As such, understanding stakeholder perspectives including patients must be central when translating this technology from the lab to the clinic. Additionally, future studies should also provide greater feedback from the users of BCI devices. In particular, the ease of use and the mental effort that is required is often missed in many studies. This will provide great insight into the rehabilitation process that is required during the post-implantation period and can provide a useful learning area for other researchers to benefit from. Having user interfaces or integrated AI modalities that make it easier for users to engage with the BCI can be as useful as improving the technical designs of the BCIs in improving patient outcomes.

User feedback is rarely reported in detail in these studies. Whilst some studies allude to improved user experience—for example, with an easier-to-use keyboard, feedback mechanism, or improved calibration strategies—a qualitative study that assesses the user experience is necessary to explore this in more depth, which includes the complete rehabilitation phase from the post-operative phase to chronic implantation. This will allow a greater understanding of the patient experience and can be used in conjunction with objective markers such as characters per minute, the speed of character selection, and recovery times.

To effectively compare studies, there needs to be homogeneity in protocol design and reporting outcomes in patients.

7. Limitations

There are several limitations to this study. A scoping review cannot guarantee that all studies assessing intracortical BCIs for communication are exhausted, found and analysed. The literature output is confined by the search terms that we entered, and although we attempted to keep the search terms as broad as possible, it is possible that relevant studies were missed out. This includes studies that have labelled their devices as anything other than a 'brain–computer interface'. The focus of this scoping review was on patients suffering from the disease as opposed to healthy participants; indeed, to our knowledge there are no invasive systems being tested on non-impaired individuals. Due to the small sample size, statistical analysis was difficult to conduct. It is also important to acknowledge that there are likely multiple user factors that affect the accuracy of signal translation, making it difficult to draw meaningful conclusions that can be applied to all patients with these conditions.

Author Contributions: Conceptualization, S.K. and A.K.; methodology, S.K. and S.E.H.; software, S.K.; investigation, S.K.; data curation, S.K. and L.K.; writing—original draft preparation, S.K. and L.K.; writing—review and editing, S.K., A.K., S.E.H., D.B. and H.M.; supervision, A.K. and P.H. All authors have read and agreed to the published version of the manuscript.

Funding: This research was funded by the NIHR ref: NIHR132455 using UK aid from the UK Government to support global health research. The views expressed in this publication are those of the authors and not necessarily those of the NIHR or the UK government. H.M. is supported by the NIHR (Health Technology Assessment program). P.H. is supported by the NIHR (Senior Investigator Award, Cambridge BRC, NIHR HRC for Brain Injury) and the Royal College of Surgeons of England. A.K. is supported by the NIHR (Cambridge BRC, Health Technology Assessment program), the Royal College of Surgeons of England and the Wellcome Trust (ISSF Fund).

Conflicts of Interest: All authors declare no conflicts of interest.

References

1. Felgoise, S.H.; Zaccheo, V.; Duff, J.; Simmons, Z. Verbal communication impacts quality of life in patients with amyotrophic lateral sclerosis. *Amyotroph. Lateral Scler. Front. Degener.* **2016**, *17*, 179–183. [CrossRef]
2. Kohnen, R.F.; Lavrijsen, J.C.M.; Bor, J.H.J.; Koopmans, R.T.C.M. The prevalence and characteristics of patients with classic locked-in syndrome in Dutch nursing homes. *J. Neurol.* **2013**, *260*, 1527–1534. [CrossRef] [PubMed]

3. Voity, K.; Lopez, T.; Chan, J.P.; Greenwald, B.D. Update on How to Approach a Patient with Locked-In Syndrome and Their Communication Ability. *Brain Sci.* **2024**, *14*, 92. [CrossRef] [PubMed]
4. Brumberg, J.S.; Pitt, K.M.; Mantie-Kozlowski, A.; Burnison, J.D. Brain–Computer Interfaces for Augmentative and Alternative Communication: A Tutorial. *Am. J. Speech-Lang. Pathol.* **2018**, *27*, 1–12. [CrossRef] [PubMed]
5. Fager, S.K.; Fried-Oken, M.; Jakobs, T.; Beukelman, D.R. New and emerging access technologies for adults with complex communication needs and severe motor impairments: State of the science. *Augment. Altern. Commun.* **2019**, *35*, 13–25. [CrossRef]
6. Oken, B.S.; Orhan, U.; Roark, B.; Erdogmus, D.; Fowler, A.; Mooney, A.; Peters, B.; Miller, M.; Fried-Oken, M.B. Brain–computer interface with language model–electroencephalography fusion for locked-in syndrome. *Neurorehabilit. Neural Repair.* **2013**, *28*, 387–394. [CrossRef]
7. Khan, S.; Anderson, W.; Constandinou, T. Surgical Implantation of Brain Computer Interfaces. *JAMA Surg.* **2024**, *159*, 219–220. [CrossRef]
8. Khan, S.; Aziz, T. Transcending the brain: Is there a cost to hacking the nervous system? *Brain Commun.* **2019**, *1*, fcz015. [CrossRef]
9. Fernández-de Thomas, R.; Munakomi, S.; De Jesus, O. *Craniotomy*; StatPearls Publishing: St. Petersburg, FL, USA, 2024.
10. Pun, T.K.; Khoshnevis, M.; Hosman, T.; Wilson, G.H.; Kapitonava, A.; Kamdar, F.; Henderson, J.M.; Simeral, J.D.; Vargas-Irwin, C.E.; Harrison, M.T.; et al. Measuring instability in chronic human intracortical neural recordings towards stable, long-term brain-computer interfaces. *Commun. Biol.* **2024**, *7*, 1–14. [CrossRef]
11. Card, N.S.; Wairagkar, M.; Iacobacci, C.; Hou, X.; Singer-Clark, T.; Willett, F.R.; Kunz, E.M.; Fan, C.; Vahdati Nia, M.; Deo, D.R.; et al. An Accurate and Rapidly Calibrating Speech Neuroprosthesis. *N. Engl. J. Med.* **2024**, *391*, 609–618. [CrossRef]
12. Silva, A.B.; Liu, J.R.; Metzger, S.L.; Bhaya-Grossman, I.; Dougherty, M.E.; Seaton, M.P.; Littlejohn, K.T.; Tu-Chan, A.; Ganguly, K.; Moses, D.A.; et al. A bilingual speech neuroprosthesis driven by cortical articulatory representations shared between languages. *Nat. Biomed. Eng.* **2024**, *8*, 977–991. [CrossRef] [PubMed]
13. Wandelt, S.K.; Bjanes, D.A.; Pejsa, K.; Lee, B.; Liu, C.; Andersen, R.A. Representation of internal speech by single neurons in human supramarginal gyrus. *Nat. Hum. Behav.* **2024**, *8*, 1136–1149. [CrossRef] [PubMed]
14. Angrick, M.; Luo, S.; Rabbani, Q.; Candrea, D.N.; Shah, S.; Milsap, G.W.; Anderson, W.S.; Gordon, C.R.; Rosenblatt, K.R.; Clawson, L.; et al. Online speech synthesis using a chronically implanted brain computer interface in an individual with ALS. *Sci. Rep.* **2024**, *14*, 1–13. [CrossRef] [PubMed]
15. Tankus, A.; Rosenberg, N.; Ben-Hamo, O.; Stern, E.; Strauss, I. Machine learning decoding of single neurons in the thalamus for speech brain-machine interfaces. *J. Neural Eng.* **2024**, *21*, 036009. [CrossRef]
16. Vansteensel, M.J.; Leinders, S.; Branco, M.P.; Crone, N.E.; Denison, T.; Freudenburg, Z.V.; Geukes, S.H.; Gosselaar, P.H.; Raemaekers, M.; Schippers, A.; et al. Longevity of a Brain–Computer Interface for Amyotrophic Lateral Sclerosis. *N. Engl. J. Med.* **2024**, *391*, 619–626. [CrossRef]
17. Wu, X.; Wellington, S.; Fu, Z.; Zhang, D. Speech decoding from stereo-electroencephalography (sEEG) signals using advanced deep learning methods. *J. Neural Eng.* **2024**, *21*, 036055. [CrossRef]
18. Luo, S.; Angrick, M.; Coogan, C.; Candrea, D.N.; Wyse-Sookoo, K.; Shah, S.; Rabbani, Q.; Milsap, G.W.; Weiss, A.R.; Anderson, W.S.; et al. Stable Decoding from a Speech BCI Enables Control for an Individual with ALS without Recalibration for 3 Months. *Adv. Sci.* **2023**, *10*, e2304853. [CrossRef]
19. Wang, R.; Chen, X.; Khalilian-Gourtani, A.; Yu, L.; Dugan, P.; Friedman, D.; Doyle, W.; Devinsky, O.; Wang, Y.; Flinker, A. Distributed feedforward and feedback cortical processing supports human speech production. *Proc. Natl. Acad. Sci. USA* **2023**, *120*, e2300255120. [CrossRef]
20. Metzger, S.L.; Littlejohn, K.T.; Silva, A.B.; Moses, D.A.; Seaton, M.P.; Wang, R.; Dougherty, M.E.; Liu, J.R.; Wu, P.; Berger, M.A.; et al. A high-performance neuroprosthesis for speech decoding and avatar control. *Nature* **2023**, *620*, 1037–1046. [CrossRef]
21. Willett, F.R.; Kunz, E.M.; Fan, C.; Avansino, D.T.; Wilson, G.H.; Choi, E.Y.; Kamdar, F.; Glasser, M.F.; Hochberg, L.R.; Druckmann, S.; et al. A high-performance speech neuroprosthesis. *Nature* **2023**, *620*, 1031–1036. [CrossRef]
22. Berezutskaya, J.; Freudenburg, Z.V.; Vansteensel, M.J.; Aarnoutse, E.J.; Ramsey, N.F.; Gerven, M.A.J.v. Direct speech reconstruction from sensorimotor brain activity with optimized deep learning models. *J. Neural Eng.* **2023**, *20*, 056010. [CrossRef] [PubMed]
23. Metzger, S.L.; Liu, J.R.; Moses, D.A.; Dougherty, M.E.; Seaton, M.P.; Littlejohn, K.T.; Chartier, J.; Anumanchipalli, G.K.; Tu-Chan, A.; Ganguly, K.; et al. Generalizable spelling using a speech neuroprosthesis in an individual with severe limb and vocal paralysis. *Nat. Commun.* **2022**, *13*, 1–15. [CrossRef] [PubMed]
24. Liu, D.; Xu, X.; Li, D.; Li, J.; Yu, X.; Ling, Z.; Hong, B. Intracranial brain-computer interface spelling using localized visual motion response. *NeuroImage* **2022**, *258*, 119363. [CrossRef]
25. Wandelt, S.K.; Kellis, S.; Bjånes, D.A.; Pejsa, K.; Lee, B.; Liu, C.; Andersen, R.A. Decoding grasp and speech signals from the cortical grasp circuit in a tetraplegic human. *Neuron* **2022**, *110*, 1777–1787.e3. [CrossRef]
26. Tankus, A.; Solomon, L.; Aharony, Y.; Faust-Socher, A.; Strauss, I. Machine learning algorithm for decoding multiple subthalamic spike trains for speech brain–machine interfaces. *J. Neural Eng.* **2021**, *18*, 066021. [CrossRef]

27. Angrick, M.; Ottenhoff, M.C.; Diener, L.; Ivucic, D.; Ivucic, G.; Goulis, S.; Saal, J.; Colon, A.J.; Wagner, L.; Krusienski, D.J.; et al. Real-time synthesis of imagined speech processes from minimally invasive recordings of neural activity. *Commun. Biol.* **2021**, *4*, 1–10. [CrossRef]
28. Dekleva, B.M.; Weiss, J.M.; Boninger, M.L.; Collinger, J.L. Generalizable cursor click decoding using grasp-related neural transients. *J. Neural Eng.* **2021**, *18*, 0460e9. [CrossRef]
29. Moses, D.A.; Metzger, S.L.; Liu, J.R.; Anumanchipalli, G.K.; Makin, J.G.; Sun, P.F.; Chartier, J.; Dougherty, M.E.; Liu, P.M.; Abrams, G.M.; et al. Neuroprosthesis for Decoding Speech in a Paralyzed Person with Anarthria. *N. Engl. J. Med.* **2021**, *385*, 217–227. [CrossRef]
30. Simeral, J.D.; Hosman, T.; Saab, J.; Flesher, S.N.; Vilela, M.; Franco, B.; Kelemen, J.N.; Brandman, D.M.; Ciancibello, J.G.; Rezaii, P.G.; et al. Home Use of a Percutaneous Wireless Intracortical Brain-Computer Interface by Individuals With Tetraplegia. *IEEE Trans. Biomed. Eng.* **2021**, *68*, 2313–2325. [CrossRef]
31. Leinders, S.; Vansteensel, M.J.; Branco, M.P.; Freudenburg, Z.V.; Pels, E.G.M.; Van der Vijgh, B.; Van Zandvoort, M.J.E.; Ramsey, N.F.; Aarnoutse, E.J. Dorsolateral prefrontal cortex-based control with an implanted brain–computer interface. *Sci. Rep.* **2020**, *10*, 1–10. [CrossRef]
32. Stavisky, S.D.; Willett, F.R.; Wilson, G.H.; Murphy, B.A.; Rezaii, P.; Avansino, D.T.; Memberg, W.D.; Miller, J.P.; Kirsch, R.F.; Hochberg, L.R.; et al. Neural ensemble dynamics in dorsal motor cortex during speech in people with paralysis. *eLife* **2019**, *8*, e46015. [CrossRef] [PubMed]
33. Anumanchipalli, G.K.; Chartier, J.; Chang, E.F. Speech synthesis from neural decoding of spoken sentences. *Nature* **2019**, *568*, 493–498. [CrossRef] [PubMed]
34. Nuyujukian, P.; Sanabria, J.A.; Saab, J.; Pandarinath, C.; Jarosiewicz, B.; Blabe, C.H.; Franco, B.; Mernoff, S.T.; Eskandar, E.N.; Simeral, J.D.; et al. Cortical control of a tablet computer by people with paralysis. *PLoS ONE* **2018**, *13*, e0204566. [CrossRef] [PubMed]
35. Milekovic, T.; Sarma, A.A.; Bacher, D.; Simeral, J.D.; Saab, J.; Pandarinath, C.; Sorice, B.L.; Blabe, C.; Oakley, E.M.; Tringale, K.R.; et al. Stable long-term BCI-enabled communication in ALS and locked-in syndrome using LFP signals. *J. Neurophysiol.* **2018**, *120*, 343–360. [CrossRef]
36. Pandarinath, C.; Nuyujukian, P.; Blabe, C.H.; Sorice, B.L.; Saab, J.; Willett, F.R.; Hochberg, L.R.; Shenoy, K.V.; Henderson, J.M. High performance communication by people with paralysis using an intracortical brain-computer interface. *eLife* **2017**, *6*, e18554. [CrossRef]
37. Vansteensel, M.J.; Pels, E.G.; Bleichner, M.G.; Branco, M.P.; Denison, T.; Freudenburg, Z.V.; Gosselaar, P.; Leinders, S.; Ottens, T.H.; Boom, M.A.V.D.; et al. Fully Implanted Brain–Computer Interface in a Locked-In Patient with ALS. *N. Engl. J. Med.* **2016**, *375*, 2060–2066. [CrossRef]
38. Jarosiewicz, B.; Sarma, A.A.; Bacher, D.; Masse, N.Y.; Simeral, J.D.; Sorice, B.; Oakley, E.M.; Blabe, C.; Pandarinath, C.; Gilja, V.; et al. Virtual typing by people with tetraplegia using a self-calibrating intracortical brain-computer interface. *Sci. Transl. Med.* **2015**, *7*, 313ra179. [CrossRef]
39. Mugler, E.M.; Goldrick, M.; Rosenow, J.M.; Tate, M.C.; Slutzky, M.W. Decoding of articulatory gestures during word production using speech motor and premotor cortical activity. In Proceedings of the 2015 37th Annual International Conference of the IEEE Engineering in Medicine and Biology Society (EMBC), Milan, Italy, 25–29 August 2015.
40. Bacher, D.; Jarosiewicz, B.; Masse, N.Y.; Stavisky, S.D.; Simeral, J.D.; Newell, K.; Oakley, E.M.; Cash, S.S.; Friehs, G.; Hochberg, L.R. Neural Point-and-Click Communication by a Person With Incomplete Locked-In Syndrome. *Neurorehabilit. Neural Repair.* **2015**, *29*, 462–471. [CrossRef]
41. Márquez-Chin, C.; Popovic, M.R.; Sanin, E.; Chen, R.; Lozano, A.M. Real-time two-dimensional asynchronous control of a computer cursor with a single subdural electrode. *J. Spinal Cord. Med.* **2012**, *35*, 382–391. [CrossRef]
42. Simeral, J.D.; Kim, S.-P.; Black, M.J.; Donoghue, J.P.; Hochberg, L.R. Neural control of cursor trajectory and click by a human with tetraplegia 1000 days after implant of an intracortical microelectrode array. *J. Neural Eng.* **2011**, *8*, 025027. [CrossRef]
43. Leuthardt, E.C.; Gaona, C.; Sharma, M.; Szrama, N.; Roland, J.; Freudenberg, Z.; Solis, J.; Breshears, J.; Schalk, G. Using the electrocorticographic speech network to control a brain–computer interface in humans. *J. Neural Eng.* **2011**, *8*, 036004. [CrossRef]
44. Krusienski, D.J.; Shih, J.J. Control of a brain–computer interface using stereotactic depth electrodes in and adjacent to the hippocampus. *J. Neural Eng.* **2011**, *8*, 025006. [CrossRef] [PubMed]
45. Kim, S.P.; Simeral, J.D.; Hochberg, L.R.; Donoghue, J.P.; Friehs, G.M.; Black, M.J. Point-and-click cursor control with an intracortical neural interface system by humans with tetraplegia. *IEEE Trans. Neural Syst. Rehabil. Eng. Publ. IEEE Eng. Med. Biol. Soc.* **2011**, *19*, 193–203.
46. Guenther, F.H.; Brumberg, J.S.; Wright, E.J.; Nieto-Castanon, A.; Tourville, J.A.; Panko, M.; Law, R.; Siebert, S.A.; Bartels, J.L.; Andreasen, D.S.; et al. A wireless brain-machine interface for real-time speech synthesis. *PLoS ONE* **2009**, *4*, e8218. [CrossRef]
47. Blakely, T.; Miller, K.J.; Zanos, S.P.; Rao, R.P.N.; Ojemann, J.G. Robust, long-term control of an electrocorticographic brain-computer interface with fixed parameters. *Neurosurg. Focus.* **2009**, *27*, E13. [CrossRef]

48. Felton, E.A.; Wilson, J.A.; Williams, J.C.; Garell, P.C. Electrocorticographically controlled brain–computer interfaces using motor and sensory imagery in patients with temporary subdural electrode implants. *J. Neurosurg.* **2007**, *106*, 495–500. [CrossRef]
49. Leuthardt, E.C.; Miller, K.J.; Schalk, G.; Rao, R.P.N.; Ojemann, J.G. Electrocorticography-based brain computer interface--the Seattle experience. *IEEE Trans. Neural Syst. Rehabil. Eng. Publ. IEEE Eng. Med. Biol. Soc.* **2006**, *14*, 194–198.
50. Huggins, J.; Wren, P.; Gruis, K. What would brain-computer interface users want? Opinions and priorities of potential users with amyotrophic lateral sclerosis. *Amyotroph. Lateral Scler. Off. Publ. World Fed. Neurol. Res. Group. Mot. Neuron Dis.* **2011**, *12*, 318–324.
51. Krusienski, D.J.; Shih, J.J. Control of a Visual Keyboard Using an Electrocorticographic Brain–Computer Interface. *Neurorehabilit. Neural Repair.* **2011**, *25*, 323–331. [CrossRef]
52. Limousin, P.; Foltynie, T. Long-term outcomes of deep brain stimulation in Parkinson disease. *Nat. Rev. Neurol.* **2019**, *15*, 234–242. [CrossRef]
53. Chow, M.S.; Wu, S.L.; Webb, S.E.; Gluskin, K.; Yew, D. Functional magnetic resonance imaging and the brain: A brief review. *World J. Radiol.* **2017**, *9*, 5–9. [CrossRef]
54. Pitt, K.M.; Brumberg, J.S.; Burnison, J.D.; Mehta, J.; Kidwai, J. Behind the Scenes of Noninvasive Brain-Computer Interfaces: A Review of Electroencephalography Signals, How They Are Recorded, and Why They Matter. *Perspect. ASHA Spec. Interest Groups* **2019**, *4*, 1622–1636. [CrossRef] [PubMed]
55. Mellinger, J.; Schalk, G.; Braun, C.; Preissl, H.; Rosenstiel, W.; Birbaumer, N.; Kübler, A. An MEG-based brain–computer interface (BCI). *NeuroImage* **2007**, *36*, 581–593. [CrossRef] [PubMed]
56. Herff, C.; Krusienski, D.J.; Kubben, P. The Potential of Stereotactic-EEG for Brain-Computer Interfaces: Current Progress and Future Directions. *Front. Neurosci.* **2020**, *14*, 123. [CrossRef]
57. Parvizi, J.; Kastner, S. Promises and limitations of human intracranial electroencephalography. *Nat. Neurosci.* **2018**, *21*, 474–483. [CrossRef] [PubMed]
58. Penfield, W.; Boldrey, E. Somatic Motor and Sensory Representation in the Cerebral Cortex of Man as Studied by Electrical Stimulation. *Brain* **1937**, *60*, 389–443. [CrossRef]
59. Roux, F.; Niare, M.; Charni, S.; Giussani, C.; Durand, J. Functional architecture of the motor homunculus detected by electrostimulation. *J. Physiol.* **2020**, *598*, 5487–5504. [CrossRef]
60. Carey, D.; Krishnan, S.; Callaghan, M.F.; Sereno, M.I.; Dick, F. Functional and Quantitative MRI Mapping of Somatomotor Representations of Human Supralaryngeal Vocal Tract. *Cereb. Cortex* **2017**, *27*, 265–278. [CrossRef]
61. Eichert, N.; Papp, D.; Mars, R.B.; Watkins, K.E. Mapping Human Laryngeal Motor Cortex during Vocalization. *Cereb. Cortex* **2020**, *30*, 6254–6269. [CrossRef]
62. Shih, J.; Krusienski, D.; Wolpaw, J. Brain-computer interfaces in medicine. *Mayo Clin. Proc.* **2012**, *87*, 268–279. [CrossRef]
63. Goss-Varley, M.; Dona, K.R.; McMahon, J.A.; Shoffstall, A.J.; Ereifej, E.S.; Lindner, S.C.; Capadona, J.R. Microelectrode implantation in motor cortex causes fine motor deficit: Implications on potential considerations to Brain Computer Interfacing and Human Augmentation. *Sci. Rep.* **2017**, *7*, 15254. [CrossRef] [PubMed]
64. Sillay, K.A.; Rutecki, P.; Cicora, K.; Worrell, G.; Drazkowski, J.; Shih, J.J.; Sharan, A.D.; Morrell, M.J.; Williams, J.; Wingeier, B. Long-term measurement of impedance in chronically implanted depth and subdural electrodes during responsive neurostimulation in humans. *Brain Stimul.* **2013**, *6*, 718–726. [CrossRef] [PubMed]
65. Swann, N.C.; de Hemptinne, C.; Miocinovic, S.; Qasim, S.; Ostrem, J.L.; Galifianakis, N.B.; Luciano, M.S.; Wang, S.S.; Ziman, N.; Taylor, R.; et al. Chronic multisite brain recordings from a totally implantable bidirectional neural interface: Experience in 5 patients with Parkinson's disease. *J. Neurosurg.* **2018**, *128*, 605–616. [CrossRef] [PubMed]
66. Pels, E.G.; Aarnoutse, E.J.; Leinders, S.; Freudenburg, Z.V.; Branco, M.P.; van der Vijgh, B.H.; Snijders, T.J.; Denison, T.; Vansteensel, M.J.; Ramsey, N.F. Stability of a chronic implanted brain-computer interface in late-stage amyotrophic lateral sclerosis. *Clin. Neurophysiol. Off. J. Int. Fed. Clin. Neurophysiol.* **2019**, *130*, 1798–1803. [CrossRef]
67. Szarowski, D.; Andersen, M.D.; Retterer, S.; Spence, A.; Isaacson, M.; Craighead, H.; Turner, J.; Shain, W. Brain responses to micro-machined silicon devices. *Brain Res.* **2003**, *983*, 23–35. [CrossRef]
68. Seymour, J.P.; Kipke, D.R. Neural probe design for reduced tissue encapsulation in CNS. *Biomaterials* **2007**, *28*, 3594–3607. [CrossRef]
69. Bjornsson, C.S.; Oh, S.J.; Al-Kofahi, Y.A.; Lim, Y.J.; Smith, K.L.; Turner, J.N.; De, S.; Roysam, B.; Shain, W.; Kim, S.J. Effects of insertion conditions on tissue strain and vascular damage during neuroprosthetic device insertion. *J. Neural Eng.* **2006**, *3*, 196–207. [CrossRef]
70. Kim, Y.-T.; Hitchcock, R.W.; Bridge, M.J.; Tresco, P.A. Chronic response of adult rat brain tissue to implants anchored to the skull. *Biomaterials* **2004**, *25*, 2229–2237. [CrossRef]
71. Sharafkhani, N.; Kouzani, A.Z.; Adams, S.D.; Long, J.M.; Lissorgues, G.; Rousseau, L.; Orwa, J.O. Neural tissue-microelectrode interaction: Brain micromotion, electrical impedance, and flexible microelectrode insertion. *J. Neurosci. Methods* **2022**, *365*, 109388. [CrossRef]

72. Turner, J.; Shain, W.; Szarowski, D.; Andersen, M.; Martins, S.; Isaacson, M.; Craighead, H. Cerebral astrocyte response to micromachined silicon implants. *Exp. Neurol.* **1999**, *156*, 33–49. [CrossRef]
73. Wexler, A. The Social Context of "Do-It-Yourself" Brain Stimulation: Neurohackers, Biohackers, and Lifehackers. *Front. Hum. Neurosci.* **2017**, *11*, 224. [CrossRef] [PubMed]
74. Partridge, B.; Bell, S.; Lucke, J.; Hall, W. Australian university students' attitudes towards the use of prescription stimulants as cognitive enhancers: Perceived patterns of use, efficacy and safety. *Drug Alcohol. Rev.* **2013**, *32*, 295–302. [CrossRef] [PubMed]
75. Koike-Akino, T.; Mahajan, R.; Marks, T.K.; Wang, Y.; Watanabe, S.; Tuzel, O.; Orlik, P. High-accuracy user identification using EEG biometrics. In Proceedings of the 2016 38th Annual International Conference of the IEEE Engineering in Medicine and Biology Society (EMBC), Orlando, FL, USA, 16–20 August 2016; pp. 854–858.
76. Clery, D. The privacy arms race. Could your pacemaker be hackable? *Science* **2015**, *347*, 499. [CrossRef]
77. Khera, M. Think Like a Hacker: Insights on the Latest Attack Vectors (and Security Controls) for Medical Device Applications. *J. Diabetes Sci. Technol.* **2017**, *11*, 207–212. [CrossRef]

brain sciences

Review

Towards a New Dawn for Neuro-Oncology: Nanomedicine at the Service of Drug Delivery for Primary and Secondary Brain Tumours

Smita Khilar [1], Antonina Dembinska-Kenner [1], Helen Hall [1], Nikolaos Syrmos [2], Gianfranco K. I. Ligarotti [3], Puneet Plaha [1], Vasileios Apostolopoulos [1], Salvatore Chibbaro [4], Giuseppe Maria Vincenzo Barbagallo [5] and Mario Ganau [1,6,*]

1 Department of Neurosurgery, Oxford University Hospitals NHS Foundation Trust, Oxford OX3 0AG, UK; smita.khilar@royalberkshire.nhs.uk (S.K.); helen.hall@balliol.ox.ac.uk (H.H.)
2 School of Medicine, Aristotle University of Thessaloniki, 54124 Thessaloniki, Greece
3 Aerospace Medical Institute of Milan "A. Mosso", Italian Air Force, 20138 Milan, Italy
4 Neurosurgery Unit, Department of Medical and Surgical Sciences and Neurosciences, Siena University, 53100 Siena, Italy
5 Department of Neurological Surgery, Policlinico "G. Rodolico-S. Marco" University Hospital, 95121 Catania, Italy
6 Nuffield Department of Clinical Neurosciences, University of Oxford, Oxford OX3 9DU, UK
* Correspondence: mario.ganau@alumni.harvard.edu

Abstract: (1) Background/Objectives: Primary and secondary brain tumours often hold devastating prognoses and low survival rates despite the application of maximal neurosurgical resection, and state-of-the-art radiotherapy and chemotherapy. One limiting factor in their management is that several antineoplastic agents are unable to cross the blood–brain barrier (BBB) to reach the tumour microenvironment. Nanomedicine could hold the potential to become an effective means of drug delivery to overcome previous hurdles towards effective neuro-oncological treatments. (2) Methods: A scoping review following the PRISMA-ScR guidelines and checklist was conducted using key terms input into PubMed to find articles that reflect emerging trends in the utilisation of nanomedicine in drug delivery for primary and secondary brain tumours. (3) Results: The review highlights various strategies by which different nanoparticles can be exploited to bypass the BBB; we provide a synthesis of the literature on the ongoing contributions to therapeutic protocols based on chemotherapy, immunotherapy, focused ultrasound, radiotherapy/radiosurgery, and radio-immunotherapy. (4) Conclusions: The emerging trends summarised in this scoping review indicate encouraging advantageous properties of nanoparticles as potential effective drug delivery mechanisms; however, there are still nanotoxicity issues that largely remain to be addressed before the translation of these innovations from laboratory to clinical practice.

Keywords: brain tumours; gliomas; glioblastoma; meningioma; brain metastases; malignant melanoma; lung metastases; breast metastases; blood–brain barrier; chemotherapy; immunotherapy; radio-immunotherapy; nanoparticle; drug delivery; antineoplastic agents; micelles; hyaluronic acid nanospheres; polymeric nanoparticles; lipid nanoparticles; magnetic nanoparticles; silica nanoparticles; zirconium nanoparticles; radiosensitisers; nanoscale immunoconjugates

1. Introduction

Conventionally, brain tumours are broadly classified into primary and secondary: the former can originate from any tissue of the central nervous system (CNS), whereas

 https://doi.org/10.3390/brainsci15020136

secondary tumours spread into the brain from elsewhere. Whereas primary brain tumours can be either benign or malignant, secondary tumours are by definition cancerous lesions. Amongst the primary tumours of the CNS, gliomas are the most frequent and devastating type [1]. Those tumours can be further classified as per their aggressiveness and extent of proliferation, according to the 2021 World Health Organisation (WHO) document, into grades I and II gliomas (low-grade gliomas (LGGs)) grade III and IV (high-grade gliomas (HGGs)) [2]. In clinical practice, the least malignant form is pilocytic astrocytoma, whereas the most malignant one is glioblastoma (GBM) [2]. While GBM accounts for the most frequent subtype of primary brain tumours, other classes characterised by various degrees of local aggressiveness, such as meningiomas, are the runners-up in terms of incidence and come up on top in terms of prevalence, reflecting the operative volumes of those lesions [3]. On the other hand, secondary brain tumours (also known as metastases) are the most common forms of brain tumours in adults, and their diagnosis is increasing proportionally to the incidence and prevalence of cancer, which has been defined as a silent pandemic by the Cancer Committee of the ACS (American College of Surgeons) (https://www.facs.org/quality-programs/cancer-programs/, accessed on 10 December 2024).

Despite the application of aggressive treatment strategies, the prognosis of brain tumours is dismal. HGGs are among the most lethal of all cancers, with a median overall survival (OS) of 14 to 20 months after optimal multimodal therapy [4]. Unfortunately, even LGGs do not boast encouraging outcomes due to the evolution to anaplasia that characterises the natural history of LGGs, leading to death within 5–10 years [5]. Clinicians struggle to predict individual patients' outcomes from other primary and secondary brain tumours due to their heterogeneity (clinically and histologically). Nonetheless, some commonalities regarding their anatomical- and treatment-specific factors have been considered by surgeon-scientists to improve the quality of neuro-oncology care offered to those patients.

In the last two decades, the advent of nanomedicine has allowed for a quicker transition of new innovations from the laboratory to clinical wards and operating rooms, a transformation that has had profound implications in neurosurgery [6]. Accordingly, this study aims at showcasing the prospective changes in our diagnostic and therapeutic paradigms for primary and secondary brain tumours. Therefore, an accurate understanding of the mainstay of neurosurgical management for these lesions is propaedeutic to presenting the new strategies brought up by nanomedicine, around which this study is centred.

2. Evolution of Treatment Modalities for Primary and Secondary Brain Tumours

The mainstay of neurosurgical treatment for brain tumours focuses on aggressive gross total resection, aiming for >95% tumour resection. An all-or-none approach towards tumour cytoreduction was demonstrated to be particularly important in GBM patients by the MD Anderson Cancer Centre Neurosurgical Group [7]. Their data concluded a statistically significant correlation between survival and >98% tumour volume resection, a correlation that is much weaker in secondary brain tumours, whose survival depends on many other factors related to the staging and response to treatment of the primary lesion.

Following tumour cytoreduction, radiation therapy with concurrent or adjuvant chemotherapy is commenced within 30 days for both HGGs and secondary brain tumours [8], while for brain metastases, the choice of adjuvant chemotherapy is highly variable depending on the WHO class and grade of the primary lesion, in HGGs the first-line treatment consists of the use of temozolomide (TMZ) [9,10] in the context of the Stupp protocol, the gold standard therapy for grade 4 gliomas. In fact, a statistically significant increase in 2-year survival can be achieved with the use of RT plus concomitant and adjuvant TMZ for GBM, from 10.4% to 26.5% according to the largest international randomised clinical trial published by Stupp et al. [10]. Nonetheless, this approach, which was so successful in HGG, does not fully translate as a treatment modality for LGG [11,12]. In their multivariate analysis, Nitta et al. [13] showed the extent of resection (EOR) to be significantly associated with progression-free survival (PFS) and OS; nonetheless, radiotherapy (RT) was not associated with better outcomes. This led to the conclusion that treatment for this class of gliomas should aim for maximal resection and continuous follow-up, with the understanding that aggressive treatment with the use of chemotherapy and RT should be reserved only for tumours carrying poor prognoses like diffuse astrocytoma or those converting to high grades.

Various shortcomings currently limit the efficacy of neuro-oncological treatments in primary and secondary brain tumours. Firstly, it should be noted that various first and secondary lines of chemotherapy are currently available for brain tumours. These include alkylating agents such as lomustine and cisplatin; anthracyclines such as Doxorubicin; topoisomerase inhibitors such as Irinotecan; and plant alkaloids such as Vinblastine. Unfortunately, all these chemotherapy classes pose challenges due to their systemic toxicity, which results from either the chemotherapeutic drugs having poor efficacy in brain penetration or their short half-life. Those aspects oblige neuro-oncologists to administer high pharmacological dosages with consequent multifold side effects (e.g., haematopoietic toxicity, hepatotoxicity, nephrotoxicity, ototoxicity, and pulmonary toxicity). Secondly, given the focus on radical resection in primary and secondary brain tumours, the efforts of the surgical community have been aimed at preserving patients' executive function postoperatively. The prospective improvement and the often transitory nature of the functional impairments caused by radical surgical interventions were initially evidenced by Talacchi et al. in a large GBM cohort [8]. For this, the push toward radical resection gave rise over time to continuous improvements in preoperative planning aimed at minimising iatrogenic insults in any patient harbouring brain lesions.

2.1. Surgical Planning and Prediction Models

For a long time, tumour localisation and the associated radiological characteristics (e.g., midline shift of ≥1 cm, subcortical positioning and insular location) have been considered significant predictors of incomplete tumour removal [8]. However, multiple surgical aids, such as the use of neuro-navigation based on functional magnetic resonance imaging (fMRI) and the use of intraoperative computed tomography (iCT), real-time intraoperative ultrasound (IoUS), and intraoperative neurophysiology (IN), have progressively emerged as game changers [14,15]. These aids for the surgical removal of the tumour have been responsible for the better rates of PFS, OS, and functionally independent survival obtained in recent years. Nonetheless, case complexity greatly influences outcomes in neurosurgery; hence, grading scales that quantify brain damage and introduce valid surgical efficacy indicators have been proposed [16]. Such tools inform clinicians about the chances of achieving radical EOR and the risk of postoperative complications; nonetheless, they are subject to ongoing refinement meant to address their shortcomings [17]. For instance, the capability to preoperatively quantify the risk of iatrogenic brain damage is outshone by the progressive improvement in our imaging modalities and surgical aids. While the grading scale proposed by Marcus et al. [16] used conventional magnetic resonance imaging (MRI) to formulate predictions, Saraswathy et al. [18] demonstrated that marginal gains in surgical planning could be offered by advanced MRI sequences, such as diffusion-weighted MRI and proton MR spectroscopic imaging (^{1}HMRSI). This underscores the contribution of biomedical engineering to neuroimaging, but nanotechnology has also been demonstrated to be a potential actor for positive change. In fact, the development of high-performance contrast agents based on nanocomposites has recently received considerable attention because these new agents hold great promise and potential for more effective and safer cancer diagnosis and intraoperative visualisation of the tumour, including the presence of possible foci of disease residuals once the intended resection is completed [19]. Additionally, other prediction models, such as the one proposed by Marko et al. [20], allowed plotting the relationship between survival probability and adjuvant therapy received by the patients, putting paramount importance not only on preoperative planning and surgical management but also on postoperative treatments. This conclusion underscores the attention of the neuro-oncology community towards innovative pharmacological strategies, including those enabled by nanotechnologies, and is consistent with the grand objective of our scoping review.

2.2. *Current Strategies for Radiation Therapy*

While conventional RT following tumour debulking remains the preferred choice for GBM and uncontrollable metastatic disease to the CNS, clinicians have been advocating for a more tailored radiation therapy for brain tumours suitable for adults and paediatric cases, with the goal of reducing side effects and improving quality of life [21,22]. Stereotactic radiosurgery (SRS) is defined as a technique of closed skull destruction of a predetermined intracranial target by a single-fraction, high dose of ionising radiation using a precision stereotactic apparatus [23]; this technique boasts the benefits of minimising collateral cells' exposure to irradiation and delivers, with greater accuracy, high ablative doses centrally to the target margin [24]. SRS comes in many different forms, depending on the type of penetrating radiation utilised, Gamma Knife, Linear Accelerators, etc. [24–26]. These techniques can prove to be quite advantageous for small tumours (<3 cm^3), either alone or in combination with other surgical and endovascular treatments. In fact, SRS can also be used as a primary treatment for various primary tumours, such as meningiomas in which a 5-year tumour control rate of 85–100% has been demonstrated [27–29], as well as brain metastases. That said, even SRS is not a panacea: Gong et al. [29] highlighted that SRS using a single-fraction Gamma Knife still has limited use in tumours located close to critical intracranial anatomical structures (e.g., optic nerve, pituitary stalk, etc.) due to their radiation tolerance. To counteract this problem, scientists have investigated radiation and pharmacological strategies meant to effectively reach the CNS, protect the healthy cells in critical anatomical structures surrounding the tumour target, and prevent direct damage following ablative SRS, including long-term consequences, such as malignant transformation over time [30]. Pharmacological agents which increase the toxic effects of radiation therapy are called radiosensitisers and radioenhancers (agents which reduce the total amount of radiation required to be lethal to a given population of tumour cells) [31–33]; however, access to the CNS represents a specific challenge for any neuro-oncological treatments, and nanosolutions have been advocated for to address this specific challenge.

2.3. *Resistance of Tumour Cells to Chemotherapy*

As mentioned above, whilst chemotherapy is often indicated in the treatment of brain tumours, there are significant challenges posed by CNS penetration. However, it has also been demonstrated that over time, tumour cells develop a resistance to these chemotherapeutic agents [34–36]. One of the proposed mechanisms for this is through tumour cells' intrinsic DNA mismatch repair mechanisms and the upregulation of specific drug-resistant proteins following long-term exposure to the chemotherapeutic agent. For example, it has been described that the overexpression of the O-methylguanine-DNA methyltransferase (MGMT) protein in glioma cells leads to the inactivation of TMZ through omission of the alkyl or methyl group which is vital to its mechanism of action [34]. Similar mechanisms are in play in metastatic tumours as well. As an example, Lee et al., describe how multiple myeloma cells that are sensitised to CD40 demonstrate a marked increase in the expression of the multi-drug-resistant protein 1 (MRP1) via the AKT signalling pathway [36]. This protein then contributes to chemoresistance to Vincristine by limiting cellular uptake of the drug. The utilisation of nanoparticles for drug delivery can significantly improve drug penetration by shielding the active pharmacological substance, thus increasing its therapeutic concentrations in tumour cells and, as such, combat drug resistance, as will be further discussed.

3. Emerging Treatment Modalities Based on Nanomedicine

3.1. Overcoming the Blood–Brain Barrier Using Nanoparticles

The selectivity of the blood–brain barrier (BBB) and the blood–tumour barrier (BTB) has emerged as an important reason behind the poor effectiveness and outcomes of antineoplastic agents. The BBB is a tight barrier, formed primarily through brain capillary endothelial cells, as well as a basement membrane, that protects the brain and only allows the crossing of essential substances, such as glucose and amino acids [37,38]. Proteins such as transferrin and Lactoferrin can only cross this barrier via receptor-mediated endocytosis [37], and the passive passage through BBB is only possible for lipophilic drugs, which carry a molecular weight of less than 400 Da and eight hydrogen bonds [35]. The BTB is comprised of abnormal vessels that enclose the tumour cells and increase the interstitial pressure within the tumour microenvironment. As an estimate, 98% of small molecules and 100% of large molecules fail to achieve therapeutic levels due to a failure to sufficiently reach the brain [39], largely due to the obstacle of the BBB. Nanoparticles (NPs), on the other hand, are able to encapsulate these molecules and provide specific transportation across the BBB via specific ligands attached to their surface. These can bind to key receptors present at the BBB, hence providing the possibility of tackling previously unreachable tumours like GBMs [40]. This strategy has been proposed in various forms for enhanced preoperative and intraoperative imaging, more effective chemotherapy protocols, and safer radiation treatments [41].

3.2. Towards Nanosolutions

Nanomedicine aims at using nanostructures, possibly with biodegradable characteristics, to find new solutions to old problems: for instance, hyaluronic acid (HA) nanospheres have been suggested as BBB/BTB carriers. Attention was drawn towards HA for its immunoneutral, biocompatible, and biodegradable properties [42], which enable NPs containing HA (HA-NPs) to easily bypass the BBB due to the action of reception-mediated endocytosis, hence improving the performance of chemotherapeutics and contrast agents [42]. HA-NPs can also exert specific tumour-targeting activity, which is due to the interaction that occurs between hyaluronidases found in the extracellular matrix (ECM) and HA receptors located on the bilipid membrane of tumour cells [43]. Furthermore, primary brain tumours induce the remodelling of the ECM, and HA, which is one of its key components, has been demonstrated to increase fourfold (to levels comparable to those seen in CNS development) in primary brain tumours [42,44]. For all those reasons, Jeong et al. [45] proposed 100–200 nm HA-NPs conjugated with cisplatin to target glioma tumour cells lines. As such, they were the first research group who successfully observed an increased cisplatin release when those NPs were tested in a glioma cell line (U343MG) which releases hyaluronidases. Their proof of concept triggered further studies to test whether HA-NPs could serve as suitable antitumour carriers and delivery systems even in secondary brain tumours. To assess that, HA was successfully used to transport cisplatin, a potent chemotherapeutic and radiosensitiser [46].

The overexpression of receptors such as CD44 and RHAMM in brain tumours was another reason to consider HA-NPs. Since CD44 is a transmembrane glycoprotein and a primary cell surface receptor for HA, hyaluronic acid–ceramide (HACE)-based nanoprobes were utilised for MRI and demonstrated raised uptake of these nanoprobes in cancer cell lines with high CD44 receptor expression [47]. This showed that MRI contrast agents have greater tumour targetability when the strong affinity of HA and CD44 is exploited, suggesting that advantageous properties of HA-NPs can go beyond drug delivery systems to enhance neuroimaging protocols [47]. HA oligomers (o-HA) have also proven to be advantageous in the sense that they antagonise the malignant properties of glioma cells by competing for the endogenous HA polymeric interactions, which, as a result, interrupts HA-induced signalling [48].

This background on the applications of nanomedicine to address many unmet neurosurgical needs in the management of primary and secondary brain tumours justifies our interest in this niche of neuro-oncology. The information provided in this introductory section warrants a deeper appraisal of the scientific literature to understand how successful the harnessing of nanomedicine has been in tackling the specifics of brain tumours' microenvironment [49] and delivering innovative antineoplastic agents and immunotherapeutic, radiotherapeutic, and anti-angiogenic drugs to the CNS. Given the exploratory nature of our research quest, a scoping review represented the best way to progress forward.

4. Materials and Methods

Scoping Review Methodology

This scoping review hopes to explore recent developments in nanomedicine and its capability of delivering antineoplastic agents for the treatment of primary and secondary brain tumours. Nanomedicine as a means of drug delivery poses several advantages such as its ability to deliver poorly water-soluble drugs, its targeted drug delivery, and its transportation of large macromolecules to intracellular sites. The pharmacological targets can also be visualised in real time by integrating imaging modalities and harnessing an optically modulated delivery of therapeutic agents [50].

This scoping review was conducted in the summer of 2024 according to the PRISMA-ScR guidelines and aims to (1) identify hot topics and emerging trends in the utilisation of nanomedicine in drug delivery of primary and secondary brain tumours and (2) demonstrate whether and how nanomedicine is extending survival and quality of life in patients diagnosed with primary or secondary brain tumours.

An array of search terms was input into PubMed—National Library of Medicine/ National Center for Biotechnology Information, with the time range being set between 2010 and 2024, to find relevant articles for triaging and inclusion in this review. No language restrictions were placed on the initial search. To maximise the chances of identifying relevant trends in the management of secondary brain tumours, the most common histotypes (breast and lung cancers) and the tumour whose oncological protocols have changed the most in recent years (melanoma) were considered [51]. The following MeSH terms, and combinations of them, were therefore used: "Nanomedicine + glioblastoma + drug delivery"; "Nanomedicine + blood brain barrier + drug delivery + brain tumour"; "Nanomedicine + brain metastases + drug delivery". A flow diagram reflective of the various steps undertaken in this scoping review is presented in Figure 1.

All key statements made in this scoping review have been appropriately referenced, and a comprehensive numerical list can be found in the References section.

The Results section (Section 5) lays out all the appropriate articles that were retained for analysis in this scoping review following our initial literature search. Conflicts of opinion regarding the inclusion of any given article in this review were resolved among the authors by discussing the pros and cons through a conventional Delphi methodology (of note, this led to the exclusion of 12 articles which were not deemed relevant enough to be listed in the summative tables of this scoping review).

Data have been collected, analysed and presented in a systematic format within the main text of Section 5, as well as in the form of two summary tables presented at the end of each major subsection of the following section, where a synthesis of results is provided. Final reporting has been drafted and verified before submission against the PRISMA-ScR checklist (https://www.prisma-statement.org/scoping/, accessed on 23 June 2024).

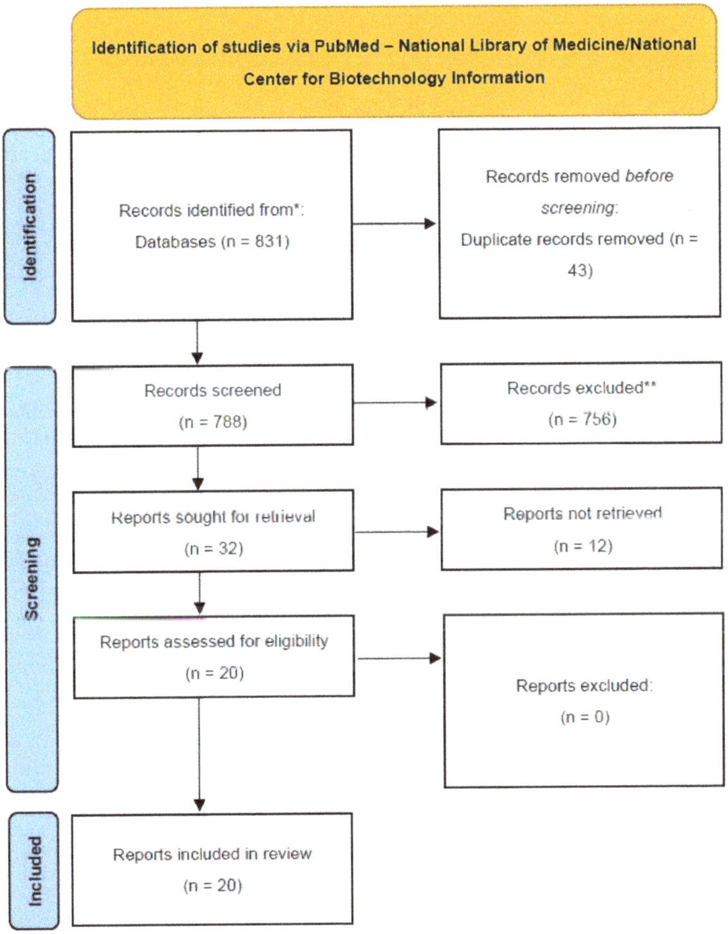

Figure 1. Flow diagram according to PRISMA-ScR guidelines, (https://www.prisma-statement.org/scoping/, accessed on 23 June 2024); * indicates that database used for the search (https://pubmed.ncbi.nlm.nih.gov/, accessed between 23 June 2024 and 31 October 2024); ** indicates all articles excluded at the time of abstract review due to either their focus (e.g., articles on the management of brain tumours not dealing with the use of nanoconjugates or articles on nanomedicine not focused or not fully dedicated to neuro-oncology) or design (non-original investigations such as case reports, editorials, and letters to editors).

5. Results

The highest number of articles (n: 657) was found when the search term "Nanomedicine + brain tumour+ chemotherapy + drug delivery" was input. Next, the search terms

"Nanomedicine + Immunotherapy + brain tumour + drug delivery" and "Brain tumour metastasis + Breast + Nanoparticle" generated 51 and 71 results, respectively. The terms "Nanomedicine + brain tumour+ antiangiogenic therapy + drug delivery"; "Brain tumour metastasis + melanoma + nanoparticle" and "Brain tumour metastasis + lung + nanoparticle" generated between 8 and 25 results. Lastly, the term "Nanomedicine + meningioma + drug delivery" only generated one result.

This scoping review highlighted various strategies exploited by different NPs to bypass the BBB and contribute to therapeutic protocols based on chemotherapy, immunotherapy, focused ultrasound, RT/SRS, and radio-immunotherapy. Those findings will be presented in the following subsections, which will cover four main areas: NPs and their various theranostics use [52–74], immunotherapy [75–140], radio-immunotherapy [141–151], and anti-angiogenic therapies [152,153]. The 20 studies retained after completion of the screening process are presented in the subsection below and summarised in Tables 1 and 2.

5.1. *The Blood–Brain Barrier and Chemotherapeutic Drug Delivery via NPs*

As mentioned in Section 3.1, the BBB can greatly limit the efficacy of antineoplastic therapeutic agents since it actively removes these agents with the means of efflux transporters like P-glycoprotein (P-gp). Paracellular diffusion is also prevented by means of tight junctions between endothelial cells [52,53]. NPs can be designed to solve this issue by encapsulating numerous drugs, bypassing the BBB and BTB, and minimising the off-target effects on the surrounding healthy tissues [52]. Targeted brain tumour nanodrug delivery can be achieved by the encapsulation of multiple pharmacological agents and by the exploitation of multiple different signalling pathways all at once. In this subsection, a dual approach will be used to summarise the evidence from the literature. On one hand, the most relevant types of NPs will be presented; on the other hand, various modalities where those NPs are used to grant passage into the CNS and tackle brain tumours will also be described. This dual approach will allow us to comprehensively cover this relevant area of nanomedicine, from strategies to increase BBB permeability, photodynamic approaches and thermotherapy, and from ultrasound-modulated chemotherapy to the use of radiosensitisers in various forms of radiation therapy.

5.1.1. Polymeric NPs

Polymeric conjugates are composed of soluble polymeric NPs that are loaded with antineoplastic agents to aid site-specific selectivity and evade processes that inhibit the efficacy of delivery of these antineoplastic agents such as protein-induced immunogenicity. In addition, these polymeric NPs can encapsulate hydrophobic drugs and increase their bioavailability.

Chang et al. [54] conjugated cisplatin with Pluronic F127-complexed PEGylated poly(glutamic acid) to produce an NP called PLG-PEG/PF127-CDDP. The NP was used on GL261 glioma cells, and a 72.53% cell invasion reduction was seen in in vitro studies. The circulating half-life of cisplatin was also increased to 9.75 h in vivo, which caused, by day 16 post-treatment, a tumour size reduction by 50%.

Annonaceous acetogenins (ACGs), a family of naturally occurring polyketides isolated from various species of the plant family Annonaceae, have been shown to have potent anti-tumour activity [55]; for instance, the monomeric component of ACG called bullatacin exhibits therapeutic activity that is 300 times that of Paclitaxel for leukaemia [56,57]. However, the delivery of ACGs is challenging due to their form being a viscous solid, making dissolution into water difficult. Ao et al. [57] used the amphiphilic polymer Poly(ethylene oxide)-b-poly(butylene oxide) (PEO-PBO) to deliver ACGs in vivo whilst also evading mononuclear phagocyte-driven NP clearance. PEO-PBO carried nanomicelles loaded with

ACGs called ACGs/EB-NCs in the following three forms: ACGs/EB_5-NCs, ACGs/EB_{10}-NCs, and ACGs/EB_{20}-NCs (depending on the ACGs/EB-NC feeding ratios). Compared to the release of free ACGs, the cumulative release rates of these three forms of ACGs/EB-NCs were significantly stronger in U87 MG cells, with ACGs/EB_5-NCs showing the highest release rate of 78.2% (within 216 h). Interestingly, though the nanomicelle ACGs/EB_{20}-NCs had the smallest cumulative release rate of 56.3% within 216 h, it showed the smallest half-inhibitory concentration and largest tumour inhibition rate.

Finally, polymeric NPs have been used for dual action on brain metastases and their primary tumours. For instance, Ashokan et al. [70] developed polymeric NPs loaded with a combination of Platin-M, a pro-drug of cisplatin, and a glycolytic inhibitor called mitochondrion-targeted dichloroacetate (DCA). In their study, the engineered nanocarrier had a terminal triphenylphosphonium (TPP) cation that could link the hyperpolarised membrane of mitochondria, which are known to be involved in ageing and carcinogenesis [112,113]. The ability to penetrate the BBB as well as the mitochondrial hyperpolarised membrane allowed the simultaneous targeting of both cancer cells located at the primary peripheral organ site, as well as those within the CNS (see Figure 2).

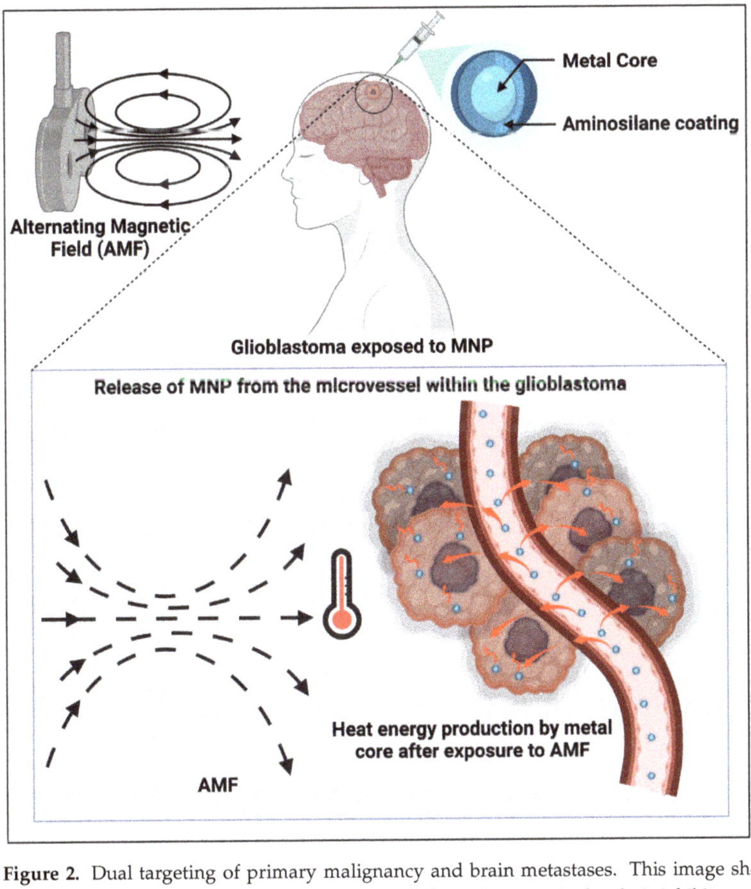

Figure 2. Dual targeting of primary malignancy and brain metastases. This image shows how polymeric nanoparticles loaded with Platin-M and chemotherapeutic glycolytic inhibitors are able to enter the mitochondria of primary malignancy in breast or lung cancers, as well as their secondary brain lesions. This approach has been proposed in breast-induced brain metastases by Ashokan et al. [70]. Created in BioRender. Khilar, S., 2025 (https://BioRender.com/d461747/, last modified on 21 January 2025).

Table 1. Summary of the studies identified which used NPs as treatment modalities for primary brain tumours. They have been divided according to the NPs serving as a delivery system for chemotherapy, immunotherapy, radio-immunotherapy, and anti-angiogenic therapy. Their administration models are also listed according to whether they were HT—a human trial; EM—an experimental model; in vivo; in vitro.

Treatment Modality Using NPs: Primary Brain Tumours	Reference	Administration Model	Strategy Described in the Study
Chemotherapy	Maier-Hauff et al. [60]	HT	Applied Intratumoural Thermotherapy using iron oxide (magnetite) NPs and alternating magnetic field (AMF).
	Liu et al. [63]	EM—in vivo (cultured C6 tumour cells) and in vitro	Combined FUS and MNPs (encapsulated iron oxide (Fe_3O_4) within poly [aniline-co-N-(1-one-butyric acid)] aniline (SPAnH) as a surface layer).
	Janjua et al. [66]	EM—in vivo (U87 and GL261 glioblastoma cell lines) and in vitro	Developed novel ultra-small (30 nm) Silica Nanoparticles for the delivery of TMZ across the BBB.
	Wan et al. [69]	EM—in vivo (Glioma cells of U251, BMSCs, HUVECs, SHG44 and U87 lines) and in vitro	Used NPs within a Zirconium-based framework to deliver TMZ with the concurrent use of ultrasound,
	Chang et al. [54]	EM—in vivo (GL261 glioma cells) and in vitro	Conjugated cisplatin with Pluronic F127-complexed PEGylated poly(glutamic acid) to produce an NP called PLG-PEG/PF127-CDDP.
	Ao et al. [57]	EM—in vivo (U87 MG cell line)	ACG-loaded nanomicelles in three different feeding ratios, ACGs/EB5-NCs, ACGs/EB10-NCs, and ACGs/EB20-NCs, were delivered using Poly(ethylene oxide)-b-poly(butylene oxide) (PEO-PBO), as an amphiphilic polymeric carrier toward U87 MG tumour-bearing mice. The NPs had the following sizes: 148.8 ± 0.5 nm, 32.7 ± 4.1 nm, and 27.1 ± 0.3 nm, corresponding to ACGs/EB5-NCs, ACGs/EB10-NCs and ACGs/EB20-NCs, respectively.
Immunotherapy	Galstyan et al. [80]	EM—in vivo (Mouse glioblastoma cell line GL261 implanted intracranially in 8 weeks old female C57BL/6J mice)	Abx against CTLA-4 and PD-1 was covalently bonded to a drug carrier called the poly (Beta-L-malic acid) PMLA backbone.
	Zhang et al. [81]	EM—in vivo (orthotopic GBM-bearing mice)	Loaded antibodies against PD-1 (as termed by the study aPD-L1) into redox-responsive micelles and combined it with Paclitaxel (PTX).
Radio-immunotherapy	Wang et al. [149]	EM—2 murine models with orthotopic GBM tumours used	Encapsulated PD-L1 antibodies (alphaPD-L1) and diselenide-bridged mesoporous silica nanoparticles (MSNs) within a mesenchymal stem cell (MSC) membrane. CC chemokine receptor 2 (CCR2) was also overexpressed on the MSC membrane. Glioma tumour cells were concurrently irradiated, which allowed radiation-induced tropism of NPs towards chemokine (CC motif) ligand 2 (CCL2).

Table 1. *Cont.*

Treatment Modality Using NPs: Primary Brain Tumours	Reference	Administration Model	Strategy Described in the Study
	Chen et al. [150]	EM—*E. coli* cells and GL261 mouse glioma cells, C8D1A mouse astrocytes, B.end3 mouse endothelial cell lines and RAW264.7 mouse macrophages	Combined gold NPs (AuNP) with an outer membrane vesicle (OMV) derived from E.Coli to create the Au-OMV complex. The complex increased ROS generation in GL261 glioma cells by 2.5-fold when they were treated with RT compared to just the Au-OMV complex alone.
Anti-angiogenic therapy	Lu et al. [153]	EM—in vivo (Orthotopic U87-mCherry-Luc glioma-bearing nude mice) and in vitro	Penetrated peptide-modified polyethyleneimine (PEI) nanocomplex with TAT-AT7 on the surface to improve binding and crossing BBB. The nanocomplex was loaded with the pVAXI-EN plasmid (secretory endostatin gene)—the total complex was termed PPTA/pVAXI-En.

Table 2. Summary of the studies identified which used NPs as treatment modalities for secondary brain tumours. They have been divided according to the tumour's primary site and NPs serving as a delivery system for chemotherapy, immunotherapy, immunotherapy + SiRNA, EGFR-tyrosine inhibitors, and radio-immunotherapy. Their administration models are also listed according to whether they were HT—a human trial; EM—an experimental model; in vivo; in vitro.

Treatment Modality Using NPs: Secondary Brain Tumours		Reference	Administration Model	Strategy Described in the Study
Chemotherapy	Breast	Lim et al. [100]	EM—in vivo (brain metastases bearing mouse model) and in vitro (BT474 cells breast cancer cell lines)	Loaded hyperbranched polymers (HBPs) with Doxorubicin (DOX) and labelled the NP with anti-HER3/anti-PEG bispecific-antibody fragments (HER3-HBP-DOX) group.
	Breast	Ashokan et al. [70]	EM—MDA-MB-231 breast cancer cell line, MDA-MB-231-BR and Breast cancer cell line HCC1806 used.	Loaded NP with a combination of Platin-M (cisplatin prodrug) and a glycolysis inhibitor to simultaneously target the primary tumour site and tumour cells that had metastasised to the brain (the potential advantages of using glycolysis inhibitors were highlighted by [112,113]).
	Breast	Liu et al. [111]	EM—in vivo (brain metastases breast cancer model)	"Trojan Horse strategy,"—a polymeric NP had a coating derived from the MDA-MB-231/Br cell membrane and was loaded with Doxorubicin. Collectively called DOX-PLGA@CM.
Immunotherapy	Breast	Sevieri et al. [107]	EM—in vitro (using D2F2/E2-Luc cells) and in vivo (murine breast tumour cell line D2F2/E2, that expressed human HER2 receptor)	Combined Transtazumab with Ferritin NPs and Docetaxel (H-TZ + Dtx) for targeted drug delivery within the tumour microenvironment and for aiding the composition of a protective microenvironment against tumour cells.

Table 2. *Cont.*

Treatment Modality Using NPs: Secondary Brain Tumours		Reference	Administration Model	Strategy Described in the Study
Immunotherapy + siRNA	Breast	Ngamcherdtrakul et al. [110]	EM—in vivo (drug-resistant orthotopic HER2+ HCC1954 tumour mouse model and HER2+ BT474 tumours within mice brains)	Co-delivery of Docetaxel and HER2 targeting siRNA via a trastuzumab-conjugated NP towards the HER2 + HCC1954 drug-resistant tumour mouse cell line.
Chemotherapy	Lung	Sambade et al. [132]	EM—in vivo (intracranial A549 tumours in nude mice)	Docetaxel and acid-labile C2-dimethyl-Si-Docetaxel (C2-Docetaxel) were carried in "Particle Replication in Nonwetting Templates (PRINT(®)) PLGA" NPs. Within A549 tumours in nude mice, median survival was seen to have increased by 35% when PRINT-C2-Docetaxel was used.
siRNA delivery	Lung	Zhang et al. [115]	EM—in vivo (mice bearing SCLC tumour metastasis model) and in vitro studies	Designed an NP capable of targeting tumour cells which had metastasised to the brain from small cell lung cancer (SCLC)—the incidence of brain metastases from SCLC is 40–50% in advanced stages of SCLC and 10% in early stages [114]. Called TP-M-Cu-MOF/siATP7a, the NP was loaded with siRNA targeting the ATP7a gene, which is important in modulating the efflux of copper intracellularly. The NP had a coating made of the TP0751-peptide-decorated stem cell membrane, which was syphilis-derived as Pallidum can traverse the BBB [120], and had a copper-based framework. Overall, the NP took advantage of cupropoptosis to inhibit tumour cell growth [116–119].
EGFR-tyrosine kinase inhibitors	Lung	Kim et al. [133]	EM—in vivo (Human NSCLC cell lines (HCC827 and H1975) and HCC827-luc cells implanted into xenograft mouse models	NUFS-sErt—a water-soluble NP designed using fat and supercritical fluid which delivered Osimertinib (a third-generation EGFR–tyrosine kinase inhibitor) for the treatment of EGFR-mutant lung cancer. This was carried out to counteract the problem of poor solubility of Osimertinib, which has been shown to have significantly higher brain penetration [138]. Significant tumour growth inhibition was seen when NUFS-sErt was inserted into the brain ventricle in intracranial xenograft model.
Radio-immunotherapy	Lung, Breast, Melanoma and Colon	Verry et al. [71]	HT—Phase I	Phase I NANO-RAD trial showing the use of a gadolinium-based NP in combination with radiotherapy for the treatment of brain metastases from breast, lung, melanoma and colon cancer.

5.1.2. Lipid NPs

Liposomes and niosomes are two examples of self-assembling concentric vesicles, which have the ability to encapsulate molecules of water-soluble, lipid-soluble, and amphiphilic nature [72]. Liposomes can also be PEGylated by the addition of polyethylene glycol chains, which can increase their half-life [72]. Further examples of lipid NPs include solid lipid NPs (SLNs), in which drugs are inserted into a lipid nucleus or core. The lipophilic nature of lipid NPs makes them a good candidate for passing through the BBB via passive diffusion or transcytosis, either receptor-mediated or adsorptive-mediated [73]. Moreover, Medes et al. describe in their in vitro study how ultra-small nanostructure lipid carriers (usNLCs) can be coupled with specific cell-penetrating peptides (CPPs), tumour-targeting peptides (TTPs), stearylamine, or transferrin, to enhance their permeability across the BBB as well as uptake into glioma cells for more targeted drug delivery [73]. Additionally, Joshy et al. demonstrated the successful uptake of zidovudine to glioma cells using modified SLNs in their in vitro study [74].

5.1.3. Magnetic NPs

The technique of enhanced permeability and retention (EPR) [58] encompasses the dilation of curved capillaries to reduce blood flow, allowing NPs to permeate through the 20–200 nm wide pores of vessels and subsequently accumulate within the tumour—these are typically sized 3–200 nm in diameter [59]. Magnetic NPs (MNPs) are advantageous due to their response to the external magnetic field (EMF) and are used for theranostic purposes (see Figure 3). Therapeutic agents can be conjugated with MNPs, and, via magnetic targeting, these MNPs can be vehiculated to the tumour site where, their local concentration can be increased to remarkably improve their therapeutic efficacy. As such, when these MNPs accumulate, their exposure to EMF causes cell destruction via heat generation [59].

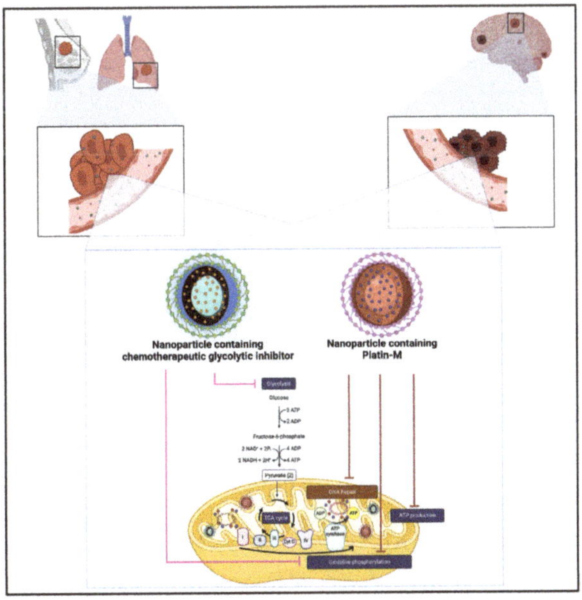

Figure 3. Intratumoural thermotherapy can be achieved by directing an alternating magnetic field towards nanoparticles containing a magnetic core. This strategy has been adopted in patients with recurrent glioblastoma by Maier-Hauff et al. [60]. Created in BioRender. Khilar, S., 2025 (https://BioRender.com/c14m563/, last modified on 21 January 2025).

A notable study by Maier-Hauff et al. [60] applied thermotherapy using an alternating magnetic field (AMF) and injecting directly into the tumour a magnetic fluid containing supermagnetic NPs, with an iron concentration of 112 mg/mL, aqueously dispersed, yielding superior responses in comparison to the standard of care [61,62].

5.1.4. Combining MNPs with the Technique of Focused Ultrasound to Increase BBB Permeability and Drug Delivery via NPs

Liu et al. [63] combined the properties of focused ultrasound (FUS) and MNPs to enhance the delivery of chemotherapeutic agents across the BBB to the tumour site while allowing for MRI monitoring during treatment. FUS reversibly disrupts the BBB and increases its permeability with the use of microbubbles and a low-energy burst tone. Due to its effects being local rather than systemic, off-target side effects are reduced. The two techniques negate the less efficient passive diffusion technique to cross the barrier due to the presence of magnetic targeting and increase the concentration of MNPs within the tumour site. The aqueous solution of the MNPs can be stabilised, for instance, by encapsulating iron oxide (Fe_3O_4) within poly [aniline-co-N-(1-one-butyric acid)] aniline (SPAnH) as a surface layer. Then, cytotoxic anti-cancer agents can be immobilised on the surface of MNPs to reduce the therapeutic quantity required. In the study conducted by Liu et al., control animals that were treated with Epirubicin-MNP without FUS had no MNP accumulation, whereas those treated with FUS/MNPs showed an estimated 15-fold higher therapeutic range of the index drug, Epirubicin, delivered to the tumour site compared to the conventional in vivo administration of a control drug, Doxorubicin (DOX). A decline in tumour volume increase was also seen; the control group had a 313% rise in tumour volume compared to the FUS/MNP group, which saw a 106 $\pm$ 24% increase. Additionally, the median survival of the group of interest was 30.5 days compared to the control group, which had a statistically significantly lower median survival of 18.3 days (p value = 0.0002).

5.1.5. Silica NPs

Although TMZ's lipophilicity and small molecular weight allow it to be absorbed orally, its BBB penetration and bioavailability in patients with GBM, or any other brain malignancies where TMZ is one of the only chemotherapy options (e.g., solitary fibrous tumours) are incredibly low at only 20% [10,62,64–66]. Additionally, TMZ has a short half-life of 2 h, and efflux pumps present within the brain tumour and BBB cause it not to accumulate sufficiently to cause therapeutic effects. This not only causes less-than-desirable outcomes, such as a 95% likelihood of GBM recurrence within 7 months of diagnosis and a <5% 5-year survival rate, but also causes drug resistance. Numerous types of NPs have been tested to optimize these shortcomings. Mesoporous silica NPs (MSNs) have been shown to exhibit properties such as a large surface area of >1000 m^2g^{-1}, excellent mechanical stability, and drug release, which can be tuned according to internal stimuli such as pH, and external stimuli, such as heat, light, and mechanical field [67,68]. This makes them great NPs for CNS-specific drug delivery systems [66]. Janjua et al. [66] developed novel ultra-small (30 nm) silica NPs with large pores (7 nm) (USLP) as a medium for chemotherapy delivery. This was combined with the Lactoferrin ligand to accommodate BBB crossing and allowed for an increased TMZ accumulation, decreased efflux ratio and improvement in the anti-cancer response [75]. Following those additional tests, Janjua et al. [66] also showed that the efflux ratio of TMZ conjugated with USLP and PEG was significantly lower than that recorded for pure TMZ (0.72 $\pm$ 0.11 vs. 2.15 $\pm$ 0.18). They also showed that when Lactoferrin as a ligand is coupled with NPs in PEG solution, it accelerates their accumulation within the brain, peaking at about 1 h post administration compared to NPs in PEG solution alone, which peak about 4 h post intravenous administration. This was estimated to be associated with the large amounts of Lactoferrin receptors expressed on the BBB.

5.1.6. Ultrasound-Modulated Chemotherapy: The Case of Zirconium NPs

Wan et al. [69] combined the beneficial properties of NPs formulated in a Zirconium-based framework (UiO-66-NH_2 NP) with ultrasound to increase the efficiency of TMZ delivery for GBM. Due to internal circulation stability, high loading capacity, and excellent biocompatibility, nanoscale metal-organic frameworks (MOFs), such as UiO-66-NH_2, provide an unprecedented opportunity for the treatment of cancer, making them an ideal drug delivery vehicle due to the superior cavity volume to load drugs such as TMZ and slow-release functions, which is expected to increase penetration through the BBB. TMZ can in fact be released through the microporous network of UiO-66-NH_2, and ultrasound accelerated this process via low-frequency oscillations. Wan et al. showed that those Zirconium-based NPs have a loading capacity of 0.25 mg of TMZ per mg of UiO-66-NH_2. Their study reflected good delivery and enrichment of the TMZ-carrying NPs locally; however, those MOFs loaded with TMZ were not able without ultrasound to inhibit tumour cell migration. The authors explained two possible mechanisms for this dismal result: either the loaded drug's release is facilitated by the destruction of the carrier, or ultrasound induces changes in the structure of the cells so that the therapeutic agent can reach the local tumour in a targeted manner.

5.1.7. NPs as Radiosensitisers

A Phase I trial called the NANO-RAD [71] trial was conducted on patients with brain metastases who were unsuitable to receive SRS. A novel gadolinium-based 5 nm NP called Activation by Guidance of Irradiation by X-ray (AGuIX) was used with RT on a total of 15 patients with 354 metastases from melanoma, lung, breast, melanoma, and colon cancer. Enhancement on MRI revealed AGuIX to have been distributed across all brain metastases. The median OS and PFS were 5.5 months. Survival 12 months after the end of the study was seen in five patients. AGuIX was also observed to be retained within the tumour for up to one week, supporting its use as a radiosensitiser and potential to be studied in Phase II trials.

5.2. *Immunotherapy*

Although several clinical trials have been conducted and others are still ongoing to test the impact of immunotherapy in the treatment of patients with primary and secondary brain tumours [75], one point that clearly emerged in all these investigations consists of the limitations of new antibody-based drugs to bypass BBB due to their molecular weight and charge. Immunotherapies exploit antigen–antibody interactions and are meant to trigger an immune response against tumours. Peptides (amino acid chains), polysaccharides (chains of simple sugars), lipids, or nucleic acids displayed over the cell membrane of tumour cells can be targeted to tackle tumour growth. In such scenarios, antibodies and aptamers, consisting of short single-stranded DNA or RNA oligonucleotides, are used to target cancer-specific molecules with high affinity in a three-dimensional shape and unchain immune reaction against primary and secondary brain tumours [140]. Given the above, in this subsection, we will cover the use of nanoscale immunoconjugates, immune checkpoints blockade, multiplexing targeting, and use of SiRNA to modulate immunotherapy for brain tumours.

5.2.1. Nanoscale Immunoconjugates (NICs)

The immune system is extremely complex and requires fine-tuning to ensure the protection of the human body. Immune checkpoints are proteins meant to keep our immune system in check, hence avoiding episodes of autoimmunity; nonetheless, they may also prevent an effective response against cancer cells, for instance, by stopping T cells from killing tumour cells in the body [84]. Regulatory T-cells (Tregs) are suppressed, and cytotoxic T-lymphocytes (CTLs), which enact an anti-tumour immune response, are activated with the use of humanised monoclonal antibodies (mAbs). Key examples of these mAbs directed against immune checkpoints are Ipilimumab, Pembrolizumab and Nivolumab, where the Ipilimumab targets the cytotoxic T-lymphocyte-associated antigens (CTLA1-4), whereas the other two drugs target the programmed cell death-1 (PD-1) pathway [76,77]. The interaction between PD-1 and its two ligands (PD-L1 and PD-L2) causes a reduction in the effector T-cell activity by inhibiting the T-cell activation via the kinase-signalling pathway, leading to immunosuppression [85,86]. Checkpoint blockade immunotherapy using antibodies against PD-1 and PD-L1 can block immunosuppressive pathways regulating the T-cells, leading to the enhancement of antitumour immune responses [63]. Hence, neuro-oncologists have tried to replicate the clinical successes obtained when antibodies targeted against PD-1 or its ligands were used to treat immunogenic tumours such as melanomas, renal cell carcinomas, bladder cancer, Hodgkin's lymphoma, and non-small-cell lung cancer [87–92]. The current body of evidence shows an in vitro lack of efficiency by these mAbs when they are administered systemically in glioma murine models [78,79]. Similarly to the strategy adopted for most NPs discussed above, to counteract the issue of antibodies not being able to cross the BBB, Galstyan et al. [80] designed an NIC, where antibodies against CTLA-4 and PD-1 were covalently bonded to a drug carrier called the poly (Beta-L-malic acid) PMLA backbone. These NICs cross the BBB and reach brain tumours using transcytosis mediated by transferrin receptors (see also Section 5.2.3). When antibodies against CTLA-4 and PF-1 were administered intravenously, after 4 and 6 h, they were barely detectable outside of blood vessels. In contrast, when they were delivered via NICs, they were detectable within the tumour parenchyma only (but not elsewhere in the brain) within 4 h. This led to the deduction that NICs hold the ability to cross the BBB and selectively accumulate within brain tumours. The survival of mice with GBMs that were treated with these NICs containing a combination of antibodies against CTLA-4 and PD-1 was significantly longer compared to when free antibodies targeted against these immune checkpoint inhibitors were administered or if only a single checkpoint inhibitor was targeted.

5.2.2. Co-Encapsulating Paclitaxel with Immune Checkpoint Inhibitors

Zhang et al. [81] also looked at antibodies against PD-1, but the innovative approach in their study was that they loaded those antibodies against PD-1 (aPD-L1) into redox-responsive micelles and combined them with Paclitaxel (PTX), a chemotherapeutic drug. The combination of antibody and the chemotherapeutic agent in a nano-micelle with angio-pep2 (A2) peptide was termed A2 APM by the investigators.

T-lymphocyte activation, the production of damage-associated molecular patterns (DAMPs) by dying cells, and dendritic cell maturation are phenomena that have been linked with immune cell death due to chemotherapy [82,83]. The point of interest here is the activation of T-lymphocytes. This combination allowed the micelles to penetrate the BTB: using an in vitro BTB model, the study showed that the utilisation of A2 peptide allowed aPD-L1 nano-micelles to cross the cell monolayers. They also showed a greater half-life for A2APM compared to free aPD-L1 (33.05 h and 23.86 h, respectively), which was noted to be associated with decreased aPD-L1 clearance as they were in a PEG shell.

Accumulation testing was carried out via aPD-L1 labelling with Cy7.5 dye. After A2APM, free aPD-L1 and APM samples were intravenously administered, and it was seen that A2APM accumulated in greater amounts 72 h post administration compared to the other groups with statistical significance. The A2APM combination also showed significant tumour regression after day 7 and 60% of A2APM mice bearing the GL261 tumour line had a striking reduction in their tumour size, exhibiting superior tumour regression properties in comparison to mice, which were treated with free-PTX, A2AM, and A2PM. The authors suggested that those latter groups were not able to elicit a strong tumour regression response due to inadequate brain accumulation.

The improved survival of the A2APM group, in comparison to free aPD-L1 and free PTX, was further explored post-resection of the gliomas: mice injected with A2APM after having their GBM tumours surgically removed under a microscope did not show any infiltrating tumour cells around the resection site or elsewhere in the rest of the normal brain parenchyma, whereas mice who received free aPD-L1, free PTX, and APM all had infiltration by tumour cells within the brain.

5.2.3. Immunotherapy with Multiplexing Targeting

The development of brain metastases can affect between 8 and 10% of adults with cancer [93]. Primary tumours from the breast and lung and melanoma contribute to the formation of most of these brain metastases [51,94]. Brain metastases from breast cancer are often diagnosed late, as only when the disease burden is significant do neurological symptoms manifest [95,154].

Human epidermal growth factor receptor (HER) overexpression is a biological signature of breast cancer, as this oncogenic receptor is also implicated with apoptosis avoidance and drug resistance via the coupling with the PI3K/Akt cell-signalling pathway [96–99]. Lim et al. [100] loaded hyperbranched polymers (HBPs) with DOX, and, to achieve tumour targeting, labelled the NP with anti-HER3/anti-PEG bispecific antibody fragments. This served as one of the first attempts to use nanotechnology to refine immunotherapy strategies for brain metastases. However, the treatment of brain metastases secondary to breast cancer can be challenging despite the use of Trastuzumab (TZ), an anti-HER2 antibody that has been shown to ameliorate patients' survival; in fact, TZ has poor penetrance to the CNS [101–103].

As seen in previous paragraphs, NPs have been used to bypass BBB, and with regard to metastatic lesions, one of the proposed strategies revolved around ferritin NPs (HFn) binding to the transferrin receptor 1 (TfR1) [104–106]. Sevieri et al. [107] conjugated TZ and HFn to compose an NP, termed H-TZ, which could specifically target HER2, as well as the TfR1 (see Figure 4).

When these H-TZ NPs were combined with Docetaxel (H-TZ + Dtx) in murine models, a statistically significant reduction in tumour growth was observed 7 days after tumour implantation in the treatment group compared to the mice group treated only by Docetaxel. Compared to free TZ, the accumulation of H-TZ within the tumour was significantly greater as per their immunofluorescence signal intensity. Impressively, H-TZ + Dtx also showed more uniform distribution on the membrane of the cancer cells compared to free TZ, further confirming that it has properties of accurately targeting the HER2+ tumour cells. It was also found that in mice treated with H-TZ + Dtx, a significant reduction in tumour development was linked to macrophage activation around tumours, suggesting that targeted TZ accumulation helped shape an anti-tumoural microenvironment. Such mechanisms are likely driven by macrophage activation post interaction between their receptors and the antibodies bound to cells, which then trigger cancer cell killing in an antibody-dependent fashion [108,109].

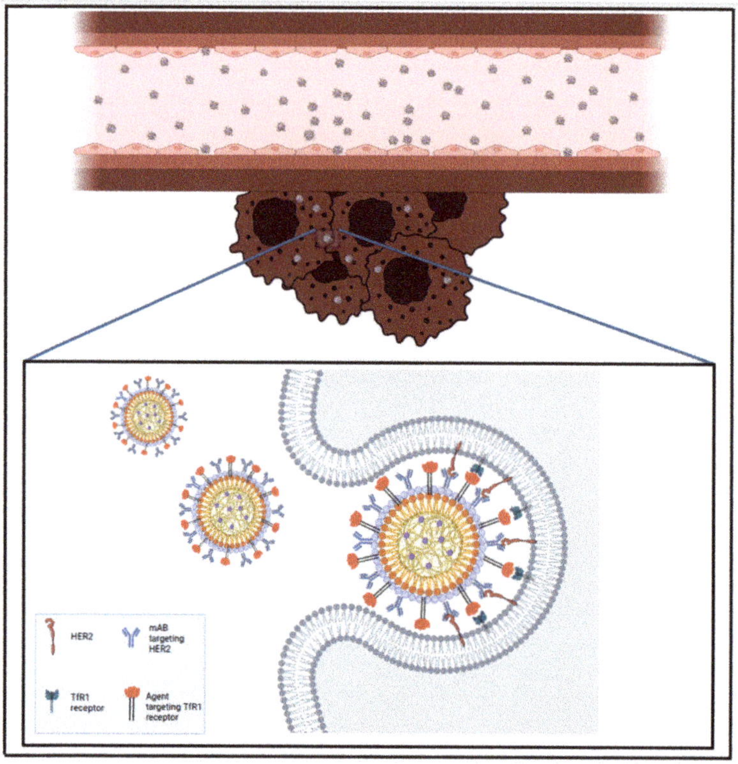

Figure 4. Immunotherapy can exploit targeted drug delivery to induce a tumour-hostile microenvironment. This approach has been used by Sevieri et al. [107] to create ferritin nanoparticles able to target HER2 and TfR1 receptors on the surface of tumour cell membranes and penetrate those cancer cells via receptor-mediated transcytosis. Created in BioRender. Khilar, S., 2025 (https://BioRender.com/c82g636/, last modified on 21 January 2025).

5.2.4. Immunotherapy Plus siRNA

Sevieri et al. [107] already showed the effective inhibition of tumour growth when a combination of TZ and Docetaxel is used and delivered via NPs. However, Ngamcherdtrakul et al., 2022 [110], combined these two agents with a siRNA against HER2 using a hydrodynamic 100 nm NP. When tested on the HER2 + HCC1954 drug-resistant tumour mouse cell line, significant tumour growth inhibition was seen when compared to the delivery of free Docetaxel. Similarly, tumour growth inhibition was seen when tested on HER2 + BT474 tumours in mice brains—however, to increase the effectiveness of NP uptake, microbubble-assisted ultrasound-guided BBB disruption was utilised. They noted the peak inhibition of the tumour occurred around day 53 post-treatment commencement and had a median survival time of 80 days compared to 54 days, when the NP was delivered without focused ultrasound.

In neuro-oncology, the term "Trojan Horse strategy" is commonly used to describe the use of receptor-mediated transcytosis (see Figure 5); this approach can be mediated by transferrin (see above in Sections 5.1.3 and 5.2.3) but also apolipoprotein [137] and photoactivated therapy candidates, such as cyclic ruthenium–peptide conjugates [138]. Liu et al. [111] referred to this masking strategy when they proposed the preparation of DOX-loaded polymeric NPs, which had a coating derived from the MDA-MB-231/Br cell membrane, "a brain homing MDA-MB-231 breast cancer cell"; collectively, their NPs were called DOX-PLGA@CM. Kaplan–Meier survival analyses showed that the systemic administration of these NPs significantly increased the survival of mice to 59 days compared to free DOX (48 days).

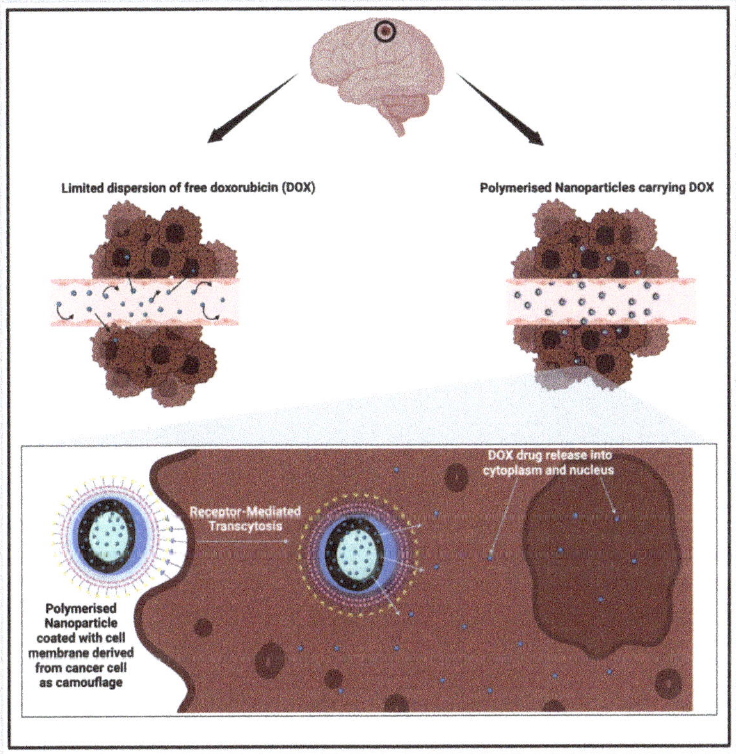

Figure 5. Receptor-mediated trancytosis can also be used to increase cancer cells' toxicity. Such a Trojan-horse strategy can be used to facilitate the release of Doxorubicin (DOX) into the cytoplasm and nucleus by nanoparticles exploiting a mimicry coating based on cancer-cell-derived membranes. This strategy has been nicely described in breast-induced brain metastases by Liu et al. [111]. Created in BioRender. Khilar, S., 2025 (https://BioRender.com/m06x929/, last modified on 21 January 2025).

Finally, the development of mRNA vaccines is giving a new boost to the hopes of finding a long-lasting treatment for various cancers. These vaccines work by encoding tumour-specific antigens and immune-stimulating molecules, effectively activating the immune system to target and eliminate cancer cells [139].

With more than 120 clinical trials to date demonstrating their potential across various malignancies, including brain tumours, nanotechnology could play a pivotal role in improving them through the mechanisms described above, hence allowing to achieve more efficient delivery and precise regulation of the immune response.

5.3. Radio-Immunotherapy

Any type of radiation therapy in principle modulates the local tumour microenvironment (TME) of irradiated lesions, a property that can be exploited with the use of immunomodulators to enhance the therapeutic value of RT [141]. In this subsection, we will explore how various nanostrategies have been used to achieve enhanced efficacy in the management of primary and secondary brain tumours; specifically, we will cover the use of stem cells, vesicles, and nanostars, and we will describe how nanomedicine helps in harnessing them against cancer cells.

In recent years, we have witnessed an increasing interest in the utilisation of immunotherapy alongside RT and chemotherapy, particularly for the treatment of HGG. Growing tumour cells/masses can prevent the body's immune cells from recognising or killing tumour cells by dysregulating signalling pathways and immunosuppressive cells or cytokines [142,143]; however, the recognition that the tumour microenvironment possesses immune privilege [144,145] led to proposing high-dose hypofractionated RT as a vital adjuvant to immunomodulatory therapy, particularly in occult metastases [141,146,147].

Going beyond primary brain tumours, Kiess et al. [148] combined Ipilimumab (Ipi) with SRS for the treatment of melanoma brain metastases and showed that the association between timing of SRS/Ipi and OS was statistically significant, and when patients received SRS during or before immunotherapy, OS was better and showed lesser recurrence of the tumour regionally. Hence, the combination of RT with immune checkpoint blockade immunotherapy has the potential to mount a robust immune response against tumour cells and potentially evade the issue of immune privilege in tumour tissue. Nonetheless, challenges still exist regarding the accurate targeting of immunomodulators to the tumour microenvironment despite synergising RT with immune checkpoint blockade therapy.

Wang et al. [149] attempted to solve this issue by encapsulating aPD-L1 and diselenide-bridged MSNs within a mesenchymal stem cell (MSC) membrane. CC chemokine receptor 2 (CCR2) was overexpressed on the MSC membrane. After irradiating the glioma tumour cells, the NPs could be directed toward the chemokine (CC motif) ligand 2 (CCL2), which is greatly expressed through radiation-induced tropism. In fact, the migration of the biomimetic nanoplatform designed in this study (which had greatly overexpressed CCR2 containing MSC), termed CCR2-SCM@MSN, was greatly improved towards the mouse glioma cell line GL261 that received X-ray irradiation pre-treatment (especially in comparison to cells that had not received X-ray irradiation).

When it came to the delivery of aPD-L1, CCR2-SCM@MSN nanoplatforms showed greater release of these antibodies and greater binding affinity when exposed to X-ray irradiation. Moreover, PD-L1 signals were substantially lost in X-ray-irradiated GL261 cells secondary to CCR2-SCM@MSN aPD-L1 exposure. Lastly, these biomimetic nanoplatforms also exhibited a reduction in immunotherapy-related adverse events by showing less colonisation with secondary antibodies in organs like spleen, kidneys, liver, lungs and heart.

The combination of immunotherapy with RT was also tested by Chen et al. [150] when they combined gold NPs with *E. coli*-derived outer membrane vesicles (OMVs), creating the complex Au-OMV. Gold NPs have numerous advantageous properties such as the ability to have numerous molecular surface coatings, biocompatibility, and ability to be synthesised into different sizes. Within the study by Chen et al., those NPs needed to have a concentration of 200 $\mu g\ mL^{-1}$ and exposure to RT to exert cytotoxic effects.

This combination also reduced the survival rate of GL261 mouse glioma cell lines (alongside B.end3 mouse brain endothelial cells and C8D1A mouse astrocytes) from 80% to 30%. Cancer cell death with the generation of reactive oxygen species with the use of metal-based NPs such as gold was already known [151]; however, this study showed that with the creation of the Au-OMV complex, ROS generation in GL261 glioma cells increased by five-fold when RT was co-applied, compared to the control group, and approximately 2.5 times the amount when Au-OMV was utilised alone.

This shows that Au-OMV complexes can serve as important radiosensitisers, similarly to the plasmonic gold nanostars [50] mentioned earlier with regard to their use as optical imaging contrast, photoactivated transducer, and therapeutic agents.

5.4. Anti-Angiogenic Therapy

The high vascularisation of brain tumours in general and gliomas in particular is the fundamental reason why anti-angiogenic therapeutics have been extremely successful as adjuvant treatments. In this subsection, we will cover how nanotechnologies have been adopted to further increase the efficacy of anti-angiogenic treatments.

Two overexpressed receptors found on the surface of new blood vessels in gliomas are vascular endothelial growth factor 2 (VEGFR-2) and Neurolipin-1 (NRP-1). In 1977, the potent antiangiogenic protein Endostatin was identified and was shown to be able to systemically inhibit tumour growth and metastasis [152]. In 2020, Lu et al. [153] designed a modified version of the penetrating peptide-modified polyethyleneimine (PEI) nanocomplex to provide a potent and safe medium of gene delivery. This was carried out by combining PEI with a dual BBB-penetrating peptide TAT-AT7 (which had been created by attaching the cell-penetrating peptide TAT to a vascular-targeting peptide AT7, to target binding to the VEGFR-2 and NRP-1) with the goal of improving the binding affinity and BBB/BTTB crossing capacity of the entire nano-complex. The combination of PEI and TAT-AT7 was termed PPTA by the study's authors, and the nanocomplex was then loaded with pVAXI-En plasmid to create PPTA/pVAXI-En. The pVAXI-EN was the secretory endostatin gene, which inhibits angiogenesis. In comparison to AT7 and TAT alone, the combination achieved a 3–10-fold greater binding affinity to VEGFR-2 and NRP-1 and exhibited a 119-fold greater endothelial cell uptake compared to AT7 alone.

6. Discussion

This scoping review allowed us to cover the vast literature on nanodrugs with the current or forecasted scope in the management of primary and secondary brain tumours. With the rapid development of delivery systems at the nano scale, consisting of either organic or inorganic nanocarriers, such as nanoshells, micelles, liposomes, and nanoparticles, it has been possible to tackle selective cancer targets relevant to neuro-oncologists. Various types of mechanisms, ranging from those to enhance BBB permeability to applications in thermotherapy, immunotherapy, and radio-immunotherapy against cancer cells, have been presented, along with the rationale for their testing in vivo and in vitro. The summary of the evidence collected through our review of the literature has then been structured in Sections 5.1–5.4 with the aim of providing guidance through this complex area of nanomedicine.

A few take-home messages should be listed.

(a) The scenarios presented illustrate the different stages of readiness, with some solutions that are already being tested in patients and others that are far too premature despite promising laboratory results.

(b) This scoping review outlines some commonalities between primary and secondary brain tumours, commonalities which can be exploited by scientists to identify innovative solutions and change the way we diagnose and treat patients with brain tumours. Furthermore, it highlights the bottlenecks of current management, from barriers to vehiculate contrast agents and drugs across the BBB and BTB to the issue of the tumour microenvironment's immune privilege [92,144,145], from metabolic plasticity for brain metastases [70,154] to the issue of nanotoxicity.

(c) We found a rising interest regarding the link between different types of primary tumours and ways to target common aspects of their biology. For instance, regarding the association between malignant melanoma (MM) and GBM, we counted fifteen studies with a total of 220 patients who all showed an association between these two tumour types [121]. Analysing those studies in detail, several mechanisms to support this linkage and possible targets for therapeutic solutions were noted, such as telomerase reverse-transcriptase promoter mutations [122–127], protein tyrosine phosphate receptor type D gene mutations occurring at high rates [128], and BRAF mutations [129–132]. Interestingly, all of them have been tested using various immunotherapy strategies [134–136], indicating that this area requires closer inspection and research, especially due to the aggressive nature of brain tumours.

It is therefore clear that various types of nanoconstructs possess specific advantages that make each of them potential valuable additions to our therapeutic armamentarium. For instance, we highlighted the ability of polymeric NPs to target brain metastases and their primary tumour, a strategic advantage that could possibly open the doors to the management not only of metastatic patients but also of those with more than one primary cancer, show are unfortunately on the rise in many worldwide statistics. We outlined how various NPs have multifold actions, from HA's ability to encapsulate contrast media and shield chemotherapeutic drugs to the specific use of magnetic NPs in adjuvant treatment thanks to their ability to be controlled remotely after administration. Furthermore, we pointed out how nanomedicine allowed diagnostic applications to be converted for theranostic purposes, moving from the intratumoural uptake of iron oxide (magnetite) NPs to their use in thermotherapy protocols (by alternating magnetic fields to provide particle heating) and fractionated SRS. These examples demonstrate not only the potential for enhancing the medical but also the surgical management of neuro-oncology patients described at the beginning of this article. All these aspects indicate a golden trend in nanomedicine, which is the tendency to identify new solutions to older problems and adopt them to exponentially increase the therapeutic options in a range of clinical scenarios.

As much as NPs often exploit their potential bioavailability and biomimicry, overall nanotoxicity remains, at present, the biggest limiting factor for the development and further application of innovative nanosolutions. Of note, the effective drug delivery provided by coating of NPs in PEG solutions (as presented in Sections 5.1.2 and 5.1.5) does not come without downsides: on one hand, this solution lacks long-term colloidal stability; on the other hand, it also exhibits high nonspecific toxicity to BBB endothelial cells. Hence, despite the advantage of providing an accelerated intratumoural chemotherapy accumulation, PEGylation strategies still suffer from a potentially detrimental iatrogenic risk. Similar risks of nanotoxicity are particularly noticeable when reviewing various NPs used for immunotherapy or as radiosensitisers. Some of these mechanisms of nanotoxicity can be unforeseeable; others can only be prevented by fine-tuning their administration. From a biological perspective, nanotoxicity can occur at the genomic (damage to the DNA per se) and/or epigenomic (alteration of the chemical and enzyme mediated processes that up- or down-regulate gene expression) level(s) and involves various direct and indirect mechanisms such as oxidative stress, inflammatory changes, the alteration of DNA replication, transcription and repair, hypoxia, the impairment of DNA methylation, histone modification, and damage to noncoding RNAs [155]. For instance, with regards to the immunotherapy strategies presented above for immune checkpoint receptors, their inherent risk consists in exacerbating immune-related adverse events due to their non-specific and systemic in vivo distribution. On the contrary, with MNPs, a precise oversight on the setting of the magnetic field (the stronger it becomes, the greater the chances of these magnetic NPs attracting one another, aggregating and causing emboli) will suffice to avoid complications.

As such, a caveat common to all the nanostrategies described above consists of the attention that should be paid by the neuro-oncological community to understand which mechanisms of actions are at play and to what extent they can generate unintended iatrogenic nanotoxicity before translating their use from laboratory settings to widespread adoption in day-to-day clinical care.

Limitations of the Study

This study has several limitations, partly due to the nature of a scoping review (which is to monitor the body of evidence on a large topic) but also related to our decision to not limit our search study to research conducted on humans. While this allowed us to describe the impact of nanosolutions on various types of tumour models, which was in keeping with our aim to review the literature on primary and secondary brain tumours, it created some heterogeneity, which we were only able to partially address when we summarised the results of our search. In practice, while the first aim of our scoping review has been achieved (to identify hot topics and emerging trends in the utilisation of nanomedicine in drug delivery for primary and secondary brain tumours), the information available to achieve the second aim (to demonstrate whether and how nanomedicine is extending survival and quality of life in patients diagnosed with primary or secondary brain tumours) was too patchy for us to achieve a conclusion. This knowledge gap justifies why we managed to explore the efficacy (explaining how and why a treatment strategy works in an experimental setting), but we failed to provide additional details regarding the effectiveness (how well a treatment strategy improves outcomes in real-life scenarios) of those nanostrategies. The ongoing development of nanomedicine discouraged us from defining strict timeframes for our search, and this increased even further the volume of articles triaged for inclusion in this scoping review. Hopefully, in our future studies, we will be able to proceed with more specific systematic review questions such as the impact of NPs on selected aspects of neurosurgical practice (e.g., intraoperative imaging, adjuvant treatment and prognostication, etc.).

7. Conclusions

Overall, this scoping review focused on identifying studies that tested and recognised the ability of NPs as potent delivery systems for antineoplastic agents that can overcome the notorious hurdle of the BBB and potentially provide a means to prolong survival in patients with CNS tumours. The results discussed indicate that the study selected for analysis focused on a variety of nanometric products aimed at use in chemotherapy, immunotherapy, anti-angiogenic therapies, and RT. These studies allowed us to evaluate, understand, and reflect on the similarities many of these strategies have, including the receptors that various NPs target, the antineoplastic agents these NPs tend to be loaded with, and the cautious strategies used to combine them all (such as for radio-immunotherapy, where a synergistic effect at delivering treatment across the BBB results in prolonging patients' survival). What we noted, however, was that several studies identified in this review worked on cell lines rather than actual human trials. This is not unexpected, considering that we did not restrict our search to translational studies but included all those with potential for future applications in human trials.

We, as authors, also acknowledge a key gap in the field—the difficulty in achieving a synergistic utilisation of several modalities into a single NP—because the tumour microenvironment possesses its immune privilege. Perhaps in the future, more studies will evaluate the plausibility of encapsulating chemotherapy agents with other immunotherapy and anti-angiogenic drugs within a single NP. Such an ideal NP could also have several specific antibodies on its outer layer to specifically target a large number of tumoural receptors.

Author Contributions: Conceptualisation, methodology, and formal analysis: all authors; writing—original draft preparation: S.K. and M.G.; writing—review and editing: A.D.-K., H.H., G.K.I.L., S.C. and M.G. All authors have read and agreed to the published version of the manuscript.

Funding: This research received no external funding.

Data Availability Statement: No new data were created by the authors of this scoping review, which has solely summarised the existing evidence from the scientific literature on nanomedicine.

Conflicts of Interest: The authors declare no conflicts of interest.

Abbreviations

ACGs	Annonaceous acetogenins
AGuIX	Activation by the guidance of irradiation by X-ray
AMF	Alternating magnetic field
BBB	Blood–brain barrier
BTB	Blood–tumour barrier
CCL2	Chemokine (CC motif) ligand 2
CCR2	CC chemokine receptor 2
CNS	Central nervous system
CPPs	Cell-penetrating peptides
CTLs	Cytotoxic T-lymphocytes
CTLA-4	Cytotoxic T-lymphocyte-associated antigen 4
DAMPs	Damage-associated molecular patterns
DCA	Dichloroacetate
DOX	Doxorubicin
ECM	Extracellular matrix
EMF	External magnetic field
EOR	Extent of resection
EPR	Enhanced permeability and retention
fMRI	Functional magnetic resonance imaging
FUS	Focused ultrasound
GBM	Glioblastoma
HA	Hyaluronic acid
HACE	Hyaluronic acid–ceramide
HA-NPs	Hyaluronic acid nanoparticles
HBP	Hyperbranched polymers
HER	Human epidermal growth factor receptor
HFn	Ferritin nanoparticles
HGGs	High-grade gliomas
iCT	Intraoperative computed tomography
IN	Intraoperative neurophysiology
IoUS	Intraoperative ultrasound
Ipi	Ipilimumab
LGG	Low-grade gliomas
mAbs	Humanised monoclonal antibodies
MGMT	O-methylguanine-DNA methyltransferase
MM	Malignant melanoma
MNPs	Magnetic nanoparticles
MOFs	Metal–organic frameworks
MRI	Magnetic resonance imaging
MRP1	Multi-drug resistant protein 1
MSC	Mesenchymal stem cell
MSNs	Mesoporous silica nanoparticles
NICs	Nanoscale immunoconjugates
NMRSA	Proton magnetic resonance spectroscopic imaging
NPs	Nanoparticles
NRP-1	Neurolipin-1

o-HA	Hyaluronic acid oligomers
OMV	Outer membrane vesicle
OS	Overall survival
PD-1	Programmed cell death-1
PEI	Polyethyleneimine
PEO-PBO	Poly(ethylene oxide)-b-poly(butylene oxide)
PFS	Progression-free survival
P-gp	P-glycoprotein
PTX	Paclitaxel
RT	Radiotherapy
SCLC	Small-cell lung cancer
SLNs	Solid lipid nanoparticles
SRS	Stereotactic radiosurgery
TMZ	Temozolomide
TfR1	Transferrin receptor 1
Tregs	Regulatory T-cells
TME	Tumour microenvironment
TPP	Triphenylphosphonium
TTPs	Tumour-targeting peptides
TZ	Trastuzumab
USLPs	Ultra-small Silica NPs with large pores
usNLCs	Ultra-small nanostructure lipid carriers
VEGFR-2	Vascular endothelial growth factor 2
WHO	World Health Organisation

References

1. Ganau, L.; Paris, M.; Ligarotti, G.K.; Ganau, M. Management of Gliomas: Overview of the Latest Technological Advancements and Related Behavioral Drawbacks. *Behav. Neurol.* **2015**, *2015*, 862634. [CrossRef] [PubMed]
2. Louis, D.N.; Perry, A.; Wesseling, P.; Brat, D.J.; Cree, I.A.; Figarella-Branger, D.; Hawkins, C.; Ng, H.K.; Pfister, S.M.; Reifenberger, G.; et al. The 2021 WHO Classification of Tumors of the Central Nervous System: A summary. *Neuro. Oncol.* **2021**, *23*, 1231–1251. [CrossRef] [PubMed]
3. Stienen, M.N.; Freyschlag, C.F.; Schaller, K.; Meling, T.; EANS Young Neurosurgeons and EANS Training Committee. Procedures performed during neurosurgery residency in Europe. *Acta Neurochir.* **2020**, *162*, 2303–2311. [CrossRef]
4. Hatoum, R.; Chen, J.S.; Lavergne, P.; Shlobin, N.A.; Wang, A.; Elkaim, L.M.; Dodin, P.; Couturier, C.P.; Ibrahim, G.M.; Fallah, A.; et al. Extent of Tumor Resection and Survival in Pediatric Patients With High-Grade Gliomas: A Systematic Review and Meta-analysis. *JAMA Netw. Open.* **2022**, *5*, e2226551. [CrossRef] [PubMed]
5. Sanai, N.; Chang, S.; Berger, M.S. Low-Grade Gliomas in Adults: A Review. *J. Neurosurg.* **2011**, *115*, 948–965. [CrossRef] [PubMed]
6. Elder, J.B.; Liu, C.Y.; Apuzzo, M.L. Neurosurgery in the realm of 10(-9), Part 2: Applications of nanotechnology to neurosurgery--present and future. *Neurosurgery* **2008**, *62*, 269–285. [CrossRef]
7. Lacroix, M.; Abi-Said, D.; Fourney, D.R.; Gokaslan, Z.L.; Shi, W.; DeMonte, F.; Lang, F.F.; McCutcheon, I.E.; Hassenbusch, S.J.; Holland, E.; et al. A Multivariate Analysis of 416 Patients with Glioblastoma Multiforme: Prognosis, Extent of Resection, and Survival. *J. Neurosurg.* **2001**, *95*, 190–198. [CrossRef] [PubMed]
8. Talacchi, A.; Turazzi, S.; Locatelli, F.; Sala, F.; Beltramello, A.; Alessandrini, F.; Manganotti, P.; Lanteri, P.; Gambin, R.; Ganau, M.; et al. Surgical treatment of high-grade gliomas in motor areas. The impact of different supportive technologies: A 171-patient series. *J. Neurooncol* **2010**, *100*, 417–426. [CrossRef] [PubMed]
9. Young, R.M.; Jamshidi, A.; Davis, G.L.; Sherman, J.H. Current Trends in the Surgical Management and Treatment of Adult Glioblastoma. *Ann. Transl. Med.* **2015**, *3*, 121. [CrossRef] [PubMed]
10. Stupp, R.; Mason, W.; Van Den Bent, M.J.; Weller, M.; Fisher, B.; Taphoorn, M.J.B.; Bélanger, K.; Brandes, A.A.; Marosi, C.; Bogdahn, U.; et al. Radiotherapy plus Concomitant and Adjuvant Temozolomide for Glioblastoma. *N. Engl. J. Med.* **2005**, *352*, 987–996. [CrossRef]
11. Duffau, H. Surgery of low-grade gliomas: Towards a 'functional neurooncology'. *Curr. Opin. Oncol.* **2009**, *21*, 543–549. [CrossRef]
12. Soffietti, R.; Baumert, B.G.; Bello, L.; Von Deimling, A.; Duffau, H.; Frénay, M.; Grisold, W.; Grant, R.; Graus, F.; Hoang-Xuan, K.; et al. Guidelines on management of low-grade gliomas: Report of an EFNS–EANO* Task Force. *Eur. J. Neurol.* **2010**, *17*, 1124–1133. [CrossRef] [PubMed]

13. Nitta, M.; Muragaki, Y.; Maruyama, T.; Ikuta, S.; Komori, T.; Maebayashi, K.; Iseki, H.; Tamura, M.; Saito, T.; Okamoto, S.; et al. Proposed therapeutic strategy for adult low-grade glioma based on aggressive tumor resection. *Neurosurg. Focus.* **2015**, *38*, E7. [CrossRef] [PubMed]
14. Ganau, M.; Ligarotti, G.K.; Apostolopoulos, V. Real-time intraoperative ultrasound in brain surgery: Neuronavigation and use of contrast-enhanced image fusion. *Quant. Imaging Med. Surg.* **2019**, *9*, 350–358. [CrossRef] [PubMed]
15. Barbagallo, G.M.V.; Certo, F.; Di Gregorio, S.; Maione, M.; Garozzo, M.; Peschillo, S.; Altieri, R. Recurrent High-Grade Glioma Surgery: A Multimodal Intraoperative Protocol toSafely Increase Extent of Tumor Resection and Analysis of Its Impact on Patient Outcome. *Neurosurg. Focus* **2021**, *50*, E20. [CrossRef]
16. Marcus, H.J.; Williams, S.; Hughes-Hallett, A.; Camp, S.J.; Nandi, D.; Thorne, L. Predicting surgical outcome in patients with glioblastoma multiforme using pre-operative magnetic resonance imaging: Development and preliminary validation of a grading system. *Neurosurg. Rev.* **2017**, *40*, 621–631. [CrossRef] [PubMed]
17. Ganau, L.; Ligarotti, G.K.I.; Ganau, M. Predicting complexity of tumor removal and postoperative outcome in patients with high-grade gliomas. *Neurosurg. Rev.* **2017**, *41*, 371–373. [CrossRef]
18. Saraswathy, S.; Crawford, F.W.; Lamborn, K.R.; Pirzkall, A.; Chang, S.; Cha, S.; Nelson, S.J. Evaluation of MR markers that predict survival in patients with newly diagnosed GBM prior to adjuvant therapy. *J. Neurooncol* **2008**, *91*, 69–81. [CrossRef]
19. Yi, Z.; Luo, Z.; Barth, N.D.; Meng, X.; Liu, H.; Bu, W.; All, A.; Vendrell, M.; Liu, X. In Vivo Tumor Visualization through MRI Off-On Switching of NaGdF4 -CaCO3 Nanoconjugates. *Adv. Mater.* **2019**, *31*, e1901851. [CrossRef]
20. Marko, N.F.; Weil, R.J.; Schroeder, J.L.; Lang, F.F.; Suki, D.; Sawaya, R.E. Extent of resection of glioblastoma revisited: Personalized survival modeling facilitates more accurate survival prediction and supports a Maximum-Safe-Resection approach to surgery. *J. Clin. Oncol.* **2014**, *32*, 774–782. [CrossRef]
21. Sanai, N.; Berger, M.S. GLIOMA EXTENT OF RESECTION AND ITS IMPACT ON PATIENT OUTCOME. *Neurosurgery* **2008**, *62*, 753–766. [CrossRef]
22. D'Arco, F.; Khan, F.; Mankad, K.; Ganau, M.; Caro-Dominguez, P.; Bisdas, S. Differential diagnosis of posterior fossa tumours in children: New insights. *Pediatr. Radiol.* **2018**, *48*, 1955–1963. [CrossRef]
23. Leksell, L. The stereotaxic method and radiosurgery of the brain. *Acta Chir. Scand.* **1951**, *102*, 316–319.
24. Ganau, M.; Foroni, R.I.; Gerosa, M.; Zivelonghi, E.; Longhi, M.; Nicolato, A. Radiosurgical options in neuro-oncology: A review on current tenets and future opportunities. Part I: Therapeutic strategies. *Tumori* **2014**, *100*, 459–465. [CrossRef]
25. Molina-Romero, O.I.; Segura-Hernandez, A.; Fonnegra-Caballero, A.; Diez-Palma, J.C.; Cortés-Muñoz, F.; Fonnegra-Pardo, J.R. Gamma Knife radiosurgery—12 years of experience in a high-complexity center of a middle-income country. *Surg. Neurol. Int.* **2022**, *13*, 582. [CrossRef] [PubMed]
26. Monaco, E.A.; Grandhi, R.; Niranjan, A.; Lunsford, L.D. The past, present and future of Gamma Knife radiosurgery for brain tumors: The Pittsburgh experience. *Expert. Rev. Neurother.* **2012**, *12*, 437–445. [CrossRef] [PubMed]
27. Apra, C.; Peyre, M.; Kalamarides, M. Current treatment options for meningioma. *Expert. Rev. Neurother.* **2018**, *18*, 241–249. [CrossRef] [PubMed]
28. Boukobza, M.; Cebula, H.; Pop, R.; Kouakou, F.; Sadoun, A.; Coca, H.A.; Polivka, M.; Diemidio, P.; Ganau, M.; George, B.; et al. Cystic meningioma: Radiological, histological, and surgical particularities in 43 patients. *Acta Neurochir.* **2016**, *158*, 1955–1964. [CrossRef]
29. Gong, X.; Ding, J.; Knisely, J.P.S.; Wang, E.; Pan, L.; Wang, B.; Zhang, N.; Wu, H.; Dai, J.; Yu, T.; et al. Dose-staged Gamma Knife radiosurgery for meningiomas: A retrospective study in a single center. *Front. Neurol.* **2022**, *13*, 893480. [CrossRef] [PubMed]
30. Imber, B.S.; Kanungo, I.; Braunstein, S.; Barani, I.J.; Fogh, S.E.; Nakamura, J.L.; Berger, M.S.; Chang, E.F.; Molinaro, A.M.; Cabrera, J.R.; et al. Indications and efficacy of gamma knife stereotactic radiosurgery for recurrent glioblastoma: 2 decades of institutional experience. *Neurosurgery* **2016**, *80*, 129–139. [CrossRef]
31. Oh, B.C.; Liu, C.Y.; Wang, M.Y.; Pagnini, P.G.; Yu, C.; Apuzzo, M.L.J. STEREOTACTIC RADIOSURGERY. *Neurosurgery* **2007**, *60*, 799–814. [CrossRef] [PubMed]
32. Ganau, M.; Foroni, R.I.; Gerosa, M.; Ricciardi, G.K.; Longhi, M.; Nicolato, A. Radiosurgical Options in Neuro-Oncology: A review on current tenets and future opportunities. Part II: Adjuvant Radiobiological Tools. *Tumori* **2015**, *101*, 57–63. [CrossRef]
33. Suh, J.H.; Stea, B.; Nabid, A.; Kresl, J.J.; Fortin, A.; Mercier, J.-P.; Senzer, N.; Chang, E.L.; Boyd, A.P.; Cagnoni, P.J.; et al. Phase III study of Efaproxiral as an adjunct to Whole-Brain radiation therapy for brain metastases. *J. Clin. Oncol.* **2005**, *24*, 106–114. [CrossRef] [PubMed]
34. Pourmadadi, M.; Shamsabadipour, A.; Bhatti, A.; Forouzanfar, M.; Rajabnejad, M.; Behzadmehr, R.; Rahdar, A.; Medina, D.I.; Díez-Pascual, A.M. Therapeutic performance of temozolomide-loaded nanomaterials: A state-of-the-art. *J. Drug Deliv. Sci. Technol.* **2023**, *85*, 104568. [CrossRef]
35. Fuchs, D.; Bley, C.R.; Morandi, L.; Tonon, C.; Weyland, M.S.; Nytko, K.J. Triple combination of lomustine, temozolomide and irradiation reduces canine glioma cell survival in vitro. *Veter. Med. Sci.* **2023**, *9*, 1573–1583. [CrossRef]

36. Lee, S.W.; Cho, H.Y.; Na, G.; Yoo, M.R.; Seo, S.K.; Hur, D.Y.; Han, J.; Lee, C.K.; Choi, I. CD40 stimulation induces vincristine resistance via AKT activation and MRP1 expression in a human multiple myeloma cell line. *Immunol. Lett.* **2012**, *144*, 41–48. [CrossRef] [PubMed]
37. Pardridge, W.M. Drug Transport across the Blood–Brain Barrier. *J. Cereb. Blood Flow. Metab.* **2012**, *32*, 1959–1972. [CrossRef]
38. Pardridge, W.M. The Blood-Brain Barrier: Bottleneck in Brain Drug Development. *NeuroRx* **2005**, *2*, 3–14. [CrossRef]
39. Zhao, Y.; Yue, P.; Yao, P.; Sun, Y.; Chen, X.; Zhao, Z.; Han, B.-J. Recent Advances in Drug Delivery Systems for Targeting Brain Tumors. *Drug Deliv.* **2023**, *30*, 1–18. [CrossRef] [PubMed]
40. Karim, R.; Palazzo, C.; Évrard, B.; Piel, G. Nanocarriers for the Treatment of Glioblastoma Multiforme: Current State-of-the-Art. *J. Control. Release* **2016**, *227*, 23–37. [CrossRef] [PubMed]
41. Leary, S.P.; Liu, C.Y.; Apuzzo, M.L.J. Toward the Emergence of nanoneurosurgery: Part III—Nanomedicine: Targeted nanotherapy, nanosurgery, and Progress toward the realization of nanoneurosurgery. *Neurosurgery* **2006**, *58*, 1009–1026. [CrossRef] [PubMed]
42. Ganau, M. Tackling gliomas with nanoformulated antineoplastic drugs: Suitability of hyaluronic acid nanoparticles. *Clin. Transl. Oncol.* **2013**, *16*, 220–223. [CrossRef]
43. Ganau, M.; Syrmos, N.C.; D'Arco, F.; Ganau, L.; Chibbaro, S.; Prisco, L.; Gki, L.; Ambu, R.; Soddu, A. Enhancing contrast agents and radiotracers performance through hyaluronic acid-coating in neuroradiology and nuclear medicine. *Hell. J. Nucl. Med.* **2017**, *20*, 166–168. [CrossRef]
44. Delpech, B.; Maingonnat, C.; Girard, N.; Chauzy, C.; Olivier, A.; Maunoury, R.; Tayot, J.; Creissard, P. Hyaluronan and hyaluronectin in the extracellular matrix of human brain tumour stroma. *Eur. J. Cancer* **1993**, *29*, 1012–1017. [CrossRef] [PubMed]
45. Jeong, Y.; Kim, S.; Jin, S.; Ryu, H.; Jin, Y.; Jung, T.; Kim, I.; Jung, S. Cisplatin-incorporated hyaluronic acid nanoparticles based on ion-complex formation. *J. Pharm. Sci.* **2007**, *97*, 1268–1276. [CrossRef]
46. Boeckman, H.J.; Trego, K.S.; Turchi, J.J. Cisplatin sensitizes cancer cells to ionizing radiation via inhibition of nonhomologous end joining. *Mol. Cancer Res.* **2005**, *3*, 277–285. [CrossRef] [PubMed]
47. Cho, H.-J.; Yoon, H.Y.; Koo, H.; Ko, S.-H.; Shim, J.-S.; Cho, J.-H.; Park, J.H.; Kim, K.; Kwon, I.C.; Kim, D.-D. Hyaluronic acid-ceramide-based optical/MR dual imaging nanoprobe for cancer diagnosis. *J. Control. Release* **2012**, *162*, 111–118. [CrossRef] [PubMed]
48. Gilg, A.G.; Tye, S.L.; Tolliver, L.B.; Wheeler, W.G.; Visconti, R.P.; Duncan, J.D.; Kostova, F.V.; Bolds, L.N.; Toole, B.P.; Maria, B.L. Targeting hyaluronan interactions in malignant gliomas and their Drug-Resistant multipotent progenitors. *Clin. Cancer Res.* **2008**, *14*, 1804–1813. [CrossRef] [PubMed]
49. Ganau, M.; Bosco, A.; Palma, A.; Corvaglia, S.; Parisse, P.; Fruk, L.; Beltrami, A.P.; Cesselli, D.; Casalis, L.; Scoles, G. A DNA-based nano-immunoassay for the label-free detection of glial fibrillary acidic protein in multicell lysates. *Nanomedicine* **2015**, *11*, 293–300. [CrossRef]
50. Yuan, H.; Wilson, C.M.; Xia, J.; Doyle, S.L.; Li, S.; Fales, A.M.; Liu, Y.; Ozaki, E.; Mulfaul, K.; Hanna, G.; et al. Plasmonics-enhanced and optically modulated delivery of gold nanostars into brain tumor. *Nanoscale* **2014**, *6*, 4078–4082. [CrossRef] [PubMed]
51. Gomez, D.; Feng, J.J.; Cheok, S.; Shah, I.; Dicharry, H.; Cote, D.J.; Briggs, R.G.; Guerra, G.A.; Peterson, R.; Salhia, B.; et al. Incidence of brain metastasis according to patient race and primary cancer origin: A systematic review. *J. Neurooncol.* **2024**, *169*, 457–467. [CrossRef]
52. Miller, D.S.; Bauer, B.; Hartz, A.M.S. Modulation of P-Glycoprotein at the Blood-Brain Barrier: Opportunities to Improve Central Nervous System Pharmacotherapy. *Pharmacol. Rev.* **2008**, *60*, 196–209. [CrossRef] [PubMed]
53. Tachibana, K.; Iwashita, Y.; Wakayama, E.; Nishino, I.; Nishikaji, T.; Kondoh, M. Tight Junction Modulating Bioprobes for Drug Delivery System to the Brain: A Review. *Pharmaceutics* **2020**, *12*, 1236. [CrossRef] [PubMed]
54. Chang, X.; Liu, J.; Li, Y.; Li, W. Pluronic F127-Complexed PEGylated Poly(glutamic acid)-Cisplatin Nanomedicine for Enhanced Glioblastoma Therapy. *Macromol. Rapid Commun.* **2024**, *45*, e2400662. [CrossRef] [PubMed]
55. Ao, H.; Wang, Z.; Lu, L.; Ma, H.; Li, H.; Fu, J.; Li, M.; Han, M.; Guo, Y.; Wang, X. Enhanced tumor accumulation and therapeutic efficacy of liposomal drugs through over-threshold dosing. *J. Nanobiotechnology* **2022**, *20*, 137. [CrossRef] [PubMed]
56. Ahammadsahib, K.I.; Hollingworth, R.M.; McGovren, J.P.; Hui, Y.-h; McLaughlin, J.L. Mode of action of bullatacin: A potent antitumor and pesticidal Annonaceous acetogenin. *Life Sci.* **1993**, *53*, 1113–1120. [CrossRef]
57. Ao, H.; Fu, Y.; Wang, X. A comparative study of PEO-PBO content on the targeting and anti-glioma activity of annonaceous acetogenins-loaded nanomicelles. *Colloids Surf. B Biointerfaces* **2024**, *244*, 114176. [CrossRef] [PubMed]
58. Maeda, H.; Nakamura, H.; Fang, J. The EPR Effect for Macromolecular Drug Delivery to Solid Tumors: Improvement of Tumor Uptake, Lowering of Systemic Toxicity, and Distinct Tumor Imaging in Vivo. *Adv. Drug Deliv. Rev.* **2013**, *65*, 71–79. [CrossRef]
59. Sindhwani, S.; Syed, A.M.; Ngai, J.; Kingston, B.R.; Maiorino, L.; Rothschild, J.; MacMillan, P.; Zhang, Y.; Rajesh, N.U.; Hoang, T.D.; et al. The Entry of Nanoparticles into Solid Tumours. *Nat. Mater.* **2020**, *19*, 566–575. [CrossRef] [PubMed]
60. Maier-Hauff, K.; Frank, U.; Nestler, D.; Niehoff, H.; Wust, P.; Thiesen, B.; Orawa, H.; Budach, V.; Jordan, A. Efficacy and Safety of Intratumoral Thermotherapy Using Magnetic Iron-Oxide Nanoparticles Combined with External Beam Radiotherapy on Patients with Recurrent Glioblastoma Multiforme. *J. Neurooncol.* **2010**, *103*, 317–324. [CrossRef] [PubMed]

61. Stupp, R.; Hegi, M.E.; Mason, W.; Van Den Bent, M.J.; Taphoorn, M.J.B.; Janzer, R.C.; Ludwin, S.K.; Allgeier, A.; Fisher, B.; Bélanger, K.; et al. Effects of Radiotherapy with Concomitant and Adjuvant Temozolomide versus Radiotherapy Alone on Survival in Glioblastoma in a Randomised Phase III Study: 5-Year Analysis of the EORTC-NCIC Trial. *Lancet Oncol.* **2009**, *10*, 459–466. [CrossRef]
62. Gubian, A.; Ganau, M.; Cebula, H.; Todeschi, J.; Scibilia, A.; Noel, G.; Spatola, G.; Chaussemy, D.; Nannavecchia, B.; Gallinaro, P.; et al. Intracranial Solitary Fibrous Tumors: A Heterogeneous Entity with an Uncertain Clinical Behavior. *World Neurosurg.* **2019**, *126*, e48–e56. [CrossRef] [PubMed]
63. Liu, H.-L.; Hua, M.-Y.; Yang, H.; Huang, C.-Y.; Chu, P.-C.; Wu, J.; Tseng, I.-F.; Wang, J.; Yen, T.; Chen, P.-Y.; et al. Magnetic Resonance Monitoring of Focused Ultrasound/Magnetic Nanoparticle Targeting Delivery of Therapeutic Agents to the Brain. *Proc. Natl. Acad. Sci. USA* **2010**, *107*, 15205–15210. [CrossRef] [PubMed]
64. Zhang, J.; Stevens, M.F.G.; Bradshaw, T.D. Temozolomide: Mechanisms of Action, Repair and Resistance. *Curr. Mol. Pharmacol.* **2012**, *5*, 102–114. [CrossRef] [PubMed]
65. Parisi, S.; Corsa, P.; Raguso, A.; Perrone, A.; Cossa, S.; Munafò, T.; Sanpaolo, G.; Donno, E.; Clemente, M.A.; Piombino, M.; et al. Temozolomide and Radiotherapy versus Radiotherapy Alone in High Grade Gliomas: A Very Long Term Comparative Study and Literature Review. *BioMed Res. Int.* **2015**, *2015*, 1–7. [CrossRef] [PubMed]
66. Janjua, T.I.; Cao, Y.; Ahmed-Cox, A.; Raza, A.; Moniruzzaman, M.; Akhter, D.T.; Fletcher, N.L.; Kavallaris, M.; Thurecht, K.J.; Popat, A. Efficient Delivery of Temozolomide Using Ultrasmall Large-Pore Silica Nanoparticles for Glioblastoma. *J. Control. Release* **2023**, *357*, 161–174. [CrossRef] [PubMed]
67. Yang, Y.; Zhang, M.; Song, H.; Yu, C. Silica-Based Nanoparticles for Biomedical Applications: From Nanocarriers to Biomodulators. *Acc. Chem. Res.* **2020**, *53*, 1545–1556. [CrossRef] [PubMed]
68. Janjua, T.I.; Cao, Y.; Yu, C.; Popat, A. Clinical Translation of Silica Nanoparticles. *Nat. Rev. Mater.* **2021**, *6*, 1072–1074. [CrossRef] [PubMed]
69. Wan, Z.; Li, C.; Gu, J.-M.; Qian, J.; Zhu, J.; Wang, J.; Li, Y.; Jiang, J.; Chen, H.; Luo, C. Accurately Controlled Delivery of Temozolomide by Biocompatible UIO-66-NH2 through Ultrasound to Enhance the Antitumor Efficacy and Attenuate the Toxicity for Treatment of Malignant Glioma. *Int. J. Nanomed.* **2021**, *16*, 6905–6922. [CrossRef] [PubMed]
70. Ashokan, A.; Sarkar, S.; Kamran, M.Z.; Surnar, B.; Kalathil, A.A.; Spencer, A.; Dhar, S. Simultaneous targeting of peripheral and brain tumors with a therapeutic nanoparticle to disrupt metabolic adaptability at both sites. *Proc. Natl. Acad. Sci. USA* **2024**, *121*, e2318119121. [CrossRef] [PubMed]
71. Verry, C.; Dufort, S.; Villa, J.; Gavard, M.; Iriart, C.; Grand, S.; Charles, J.; Chovelon, B.; Cracowski, J.-L.; Quesada, J.-L.; et al. Theranostic AGuIX nanoparticles as radiosensitizer: A phase I, dose-escalation study in patients with multiple brain metastases (NANO-RAD trial). *Radiother. Oncol.* **2021**, *160*, 159–165. [CrossRef] [PubMed]
72. Yang, B.; Yang, B.; Dong, Y.; Wang, F.; Zhang, Y. Nanoformulations to enhance the bioavailability and physiological functions of polyphenols. *Molecules* **2020**, *25*, 4613. [CrossRef] [PubMed]
73. Mendes, M.; Nunes, S.; Cova, T.; Branco, F.; Dyrks, M.; Koksch, B.; Vale, N.; Sousa, J.; Pais, A.; Vitorino, C. Charge-switchable cell-penetrating peptides for rerouting nanoparticles to glioblastoma treatment. *Colloids Surfaces B Biointerfaces* **2024**, *241*, 113983. [CrossRef]
74. Joshy, K.S.; Sharma, C.P.; Kalarikkal, N.; Sandeep, K.P.; Thomas, S.; Pothen, L.A. Evaluation of in-vitro cytotoxicity and cellular uptake efficiency of zidovudine-loaded solid lipid nanoparticles modified with Aloe Vera in glioma cells. *Mater. Sci. Eng. C* **2016**, *66*, 40–50. [CrossRef]
75. Lim, M.; Xia, Y.; Bettegowda, C.; Weller, M. Current State of Immunotherapy for Glioblastoma. *Nat. Rev. Clin. Oncol.* **2018**, *15*, 422–442. [CrossRef] [PubMed]
76. Hodi, F.S.; O'Day, S.; McDermott, D.F.; Weber, R.; Sosman, J.A.; Haanen, J.B.A.G.; González, R.; Robert, C.; Schadendorf, D.; Hassel, J.C.; et al. Improved Survival with Ipilimumab in Patients with Metastatic Melanoma. *N. Engl. J. Med.* **2010**, *363*, 711–723. [CrossRef] [PubMed]
77. Robert, C.; Thomas, L.; Bondarenko, I.; O'Day, S.; Weber, J.S.; Garbe, C.; Lebbe, C.; Baurain, J.; Testori, A.; Grob, J.-J.; et al. Ipilimumab plus Dacarbazine for Previously Untreated Metastatic Melanoma. *N. Engl. J. Med.* **2011**, *364*, 2517–2526. [CrossRef] [PubMed]
78. Wainwright, D.A.; Chang, A.L.; Dey, M.; Balyasnikova, I.V.; Kim, C.K.; Tobias, A.L.; Cheng, Y.; Kim, J.W.; Qiao, J.; Zhang, L.; et al. Durable Therapeutic Efficacy Utilizing Combinatorial Blockade against IDO, CTLA-4, and PD-L1 in Mice with Brain Tumors. *Clin. Cancer Res.* **2014**, *20*, 5290–5301. [CrossRef] [PubMed]
79. Belcaid, Z.; Phallen, J.; Zeng, J.; See, A.P.; Mathios, D.; Gottschalk, C.; Nicholas, S.E.; Kellett, M.; Ruzevick, J.; Jackson, C.M.; et al. Focal Radiation Therapy Combined with 4-1BB Activation and CTLA-4 Blockade Yields Long-Term Survival and a Protective Antigen-Specific Memory Response in a Murine Glioma Model. *PLoS ONE* **2014**, *9*, e101764. [CrossRef]

80. Galstyan, A.; Markman, J.L.; Shatalova, E.S.; Chiechi, A.; Korman, A.J.; Patil, R.; Klymyshyn, D.; Tourtellotte, W.G.; Israel, L.; Braubach, O.; et al. Blood–Brain Barrier Permeable Nano Immunoconjugates Induce Local Immune Responses for Glioma Therapy. *Nat. Commun.* **2019**, *10*, 3850. [CrossRef] [PubMed]
81. Zhang, Z.Y.; Xu, X.; Juan, D.; Chen, X.; Xue, Y.; Zhang, J.; Yang, X.; Chen, X.; Xie, J.; Ju, S. Redox-Responsive Polymer Micelles Co-Encapsulating Immune Checkpoint Inhibitors and Chemotherapeutic Agents for Glioblastoma Therapy. *Nat. Commun.* **2024**, *15*, 1118. [CrossRef] [PubMed]
82. Qi, J.; Fan, J.; You, Y.; Du, Y.; Liu, D.; Xu, X.; Wang, J.; Zhu, L.; Chen, M.; Gao, S.; et al. Synergistic Effect of Tumor Chemo-Immunotherapy Induced by Leukocyte-Hitchhiking Thermal-Sensitive Micelles. *Nat. Commun.* **2021**, *12*, 4755. [CrossRef] [PubMed]
83. Zhou, J.; Wang, G.; Chen, Y.; Wang, H.; Hua, Y.; Cai, Z. Immunogenic Cell Death in Cancer Therapy: Present and Emerging Inducers. *J. Cell Mol. Med.* **2019**, *23*, 4854–4865. [CrossRef] [PubMed]
84. Sharma, P.; Allison, J.P. The future of immune checkpoint therapy. *Science* **2015**, *348*, 56–61. [CrossRef] [PubMed]
85. Francisco, L.M.; Sage, P.T.; Sharpe, A.H. The PD-1 pathway in tolerance and autoimmunity. *Immunol. Rev.* **2010**, *236*, 219–242. [CrossRef]
86. Ansell, S.M.; Lesokhin, A.M.; Borrello, I.; Halwani, A.; Scott, E.C.; Gutierrez, M.; Schuster, S.J.; Millenson, M.M.; Cattry, D.; Freeman, G.J.; et al. PD-1 Blockade with Nivolumab in Relapsed or Refractory Hodgkin's Lymphoma. *N. Engl. J. Med.* **2014**, *372*, 311–319. [CrossRef]
87. Herbst, R.S.; Soria, J.-C.; Kowanetz, M.; Fine, G.D.; Hamid, O.; Gordon, M.S.; Sosman, J.A.; McDermott, D.F.; Powderly, J.D.; Gettinger, S.N.; et al. Predictive correlates of response to the anti-PD-L1 antibody MPDL3280A in cancer patients. *Nature* **2014**, *515*, 563–567. [CrossRef]
88. Powles, T.; Eder, J.P.; Fine, G.D.; Braiteh, F.S.; Loriot, Y.; Cruz, C.; Bellmunt, J.; Burris, H.A.; Petrylak, D.P.; Teng, S.-L.; et al. MPDL3280A (anti-PD-L1) treatment leads to clinical activity in metastatic bladder cancer. *Nature* **2014**, *515*, 558–562. [CrossRef]
89. Topalian, S.L.; Sznol, M.; McDermott, D.F.; Kluger, H.M.; Carvajal, R.D.; Sharfman, W.H.; Brahmer, J.R.; Lawrence, D.P.; Atkins, M.B.; Powderly, J.D.; et al. Survival, durable tumor remission, and Long-Term safety in patients with advanced melanoma receiving Nivolumab. *J. Clin. Oncol.* **2014**, *32*, 1020–1030. [CrossRef] [PubMed]
90. Taube, J.M.; Klein, A.; Brahmer, J.R.; Xu, H.; Pan, X.; Kim, J.H.; Chen, L.; Pardoll, D.M.; Topalian, S.L.; Anders, R.A. Association of PD-1, PD-1 Ligands, and Other Features of the Tumor Immune Microenvironment with Response to Anti–PD-1 Therapy. *Clin. Cancer Res.* **2014**, *20*, 5064–5074. [CrossRef] [PubMed]
91. Le, D.T.; Uram, J.N.; Wang, H.; Bartlett, B.R.; Kemberling, H.; Eyring, A.D.; Skora, A.D.; Luber, B.S.; Azad, N.S.; Laheru, D.; et al. PD-1 Blockade in Tumors with Mismatch-Repair Deficiency. *N. Engl. J. Med.* **2015**, *372*, 2509–2520. [CrossRef] [PubMed]
92. Shahabi, V.; Postow, M.A.; Tuck, D.; Wolchok, J.D. Immune-priming of the tumor microenvironment by radiotherapy. *Am. J. Clin. Oncol.* **2013**, *38*, 90–97. [CrossRef] [PubMed]
93. Schouten, L.J.; Rutten, J.; Huveneers, H.a.M.; Twijnstra, A. Incidence of brain metastases in a cohort of patients with carcinoma of the breast, colon, kidney, and lung and melanoma. *Cancer* **2002**, *94*, 2698–2705. [CrossRef] [PubMed]
94. Eichler, A.F.; Loeffler, J.S. Multidisciplinary management of brain metastases. *Oncologist* **2007**, *12*, 884–898. [CrossRef] [PubMed]
95. Cagney, D.; Martin, A.; Catalano, P.J.; Brown, P.D.; Alexander, B.M.; Lin, N.U.; Aizer, A.A. Implications of Screening for Brain Metastases in Patients with Breast Cancer and Non–Small Cell Lung Cancer. *JAMA Oncol.* **2018**, *4*, 1001. [CrossRef]
96. McTyre, E.; Scott, J.G.; Chinnaiyan, P. Whole Brain Radiotherapy for Brain Metastasis. *Surg. Neurol. Int.* **2013**, *4*, 236. [CrossRef]
97. Hsieh, A.C.; Moasser, M.M. Targeting HER Proteins in Cancer Therapy and the Role of the Non-Target HER3. *Br. J. Cancer* **2007**, *97*, 453–457. [CrossRef] [PubMed]
98. Barros, F.; Abdel-Fatah, T.M.A.; Moseley, P.M.; Nolan, C.C.; Durham, A.C.; Rakha, E.A.; Chan, S.; Ellis, I.O.; Green, A. Characterisation of HER Heterodimers in Breast Cancer Using in Situ Proximity Ligation Assay. *Breast Cancer Res. Treat.* **2014**, *144*, 273–285. [CrossRef]
99. Green, A.; Barros, F.; Abdel-Fatah, T.M.; Moseley, P.M.; Nolan, C.C.; Durham, A.C.; Rakha, E.A.; Chan, S.; Ellis, I.O. HER2/HER3 Heterodimers and P21 Expression Are Capable of Predicting Adjuvant Trastuzumab Response in HER2+ Breast Cancer. *Breast Cancer Res. Treat.* **2014**, *145*, 33–44. [CrossRef]
100. Lim, M.; Fletcher, N.L.; Saunus, J.M.; Reed, A.E.M.; Chittoory, H.; Simpson, P.T.; Thurecht, K.J.; Lakhani, S.R. Targeted Hyperbranched Nanoparticles for Delivery of Doxorubicin in Breast Cancer Brain Metastasis. *Mol. Pharm.* **2023**, *20*, 6169–6183. [CrossRef] [PubMed]
101. Kim, M.; Kizilbash, S.H.; Laramy, J.K.; Gampa, G.; Parrish, K.E.; Sarkaria, J.N.; Elmquist, W.F. Barriers to effective drug treatment for brain metastases: A multifactorial problem in the delivery of precision medicine. *Pharm. Res.* **2018**, *35*, 177. [CrossRef] [PubMed]
102. Rathi, S.; Griffith, J.I.; Zhang, W.; Zhang, W.; Oh, J.; Talele, S.; Sarkaria, J.N.; Elmquist, W.F. The influence of the blood–brain barrier in the treatment of brain tumours. *J. Intern. Med.* **2022**, *292*, 3–30. [CrossRef] [PubMed]

103. Abbott, N.J. Blood–brain barrier structure and function and the challenges for CNS drug delivery. *J. Inherit. Metab. Dis.* **2013**, *36*, 437–449. [CrossRef] [PubMed]
104. Fiandra, L.; Mazzucchelli, S.; Truffi, M.; Bellini, M.; Sorrentino, L.; Corsi, F. In Vitro Permeation of FITC-loaded Ferritins Across a Rat Blood-brain Barrier: A Model to Study the Delivery of Nanoformulated Molecules. *J. Vis. Exp.* **2016**, *114*, e54279. [CrossRef]
105. Fan, K.; Jia, X.; Zhou, M.; Wang, K.; Conde, J.; He, J.; Tian, J.; Yan, X. Ferritin nanocarrier traverses the blood brain barrier and kills glioma. *ACS Nano* **2018**, *12*, 4105–4115. [CrossRef]
106. Liu, W.; Lin, Q.; Fu, Y.; Huang, S.; Guo, C.; Li, L.; Wang, L.; Zhang, Z.; Zhang, L. Target delivering paclitaxel by ferritin heavy chain nanocages for glioma treatment. *J. Control. Release* **2019**, *323*, 191–202. [CrossRef]
107. Sevieri, M.; Mazzucchelli, S.; Barbieri, L.; Garbujo, S.; Carelli, S.; Bonizzi, A.; Rey, F.; Recordati, C.; Recchia, M.; Allevi, R.; et al. Ferritin nanoconjugates guide trastuzumab brain delivery to promote an antitumor response in murine HER2 + breast cancer brain metastasis. *Pharmacol. Res.* **2023**, *196*, 106934. [CrossRef] [PubMed]
108. Shi, Y.; Fan, X.; Deng, H.; Brezski, R.J.; Rycyzyn, M.; Jordan, R.E.; Strohl, W.R.; Zou, Q.; Zhang, N.; An, Z. Trastuzumab Triggers Phagocytic Killing of High HER2 Cancer Cells In Vitro and In Vivo by Interaction with Fcγ Receptors on Macrophages. *J. Immunol.* **2015**, *194*, 4379–4386. [CrossRef]
109. Richards, J.O.; Karki, S.; Lazar, G.A.; Chen, H.; Dang, W.; Desjarlais, J.R. Optimization of antibody binding to FcγRIIa enhances macrophage phagocytosis of tumor cells. *Mol. Cancer Ther.* **2008**, *7*, 2517–2527. [CrossRef] [PubMed]
110. Ngamcherdtrakul, W.; Bejan, D.S.; Cruz-Muñoz, W.; Reda, M.; Zaidan, H.Y.; Siriwon, N.; Marshall, S.; Wang, R.; Nelson, M.A.; Rehwaldt, J.P.C.; et al. Targeted nanoparticle for co-delivery of HER2 siRNA and a taxane to mirror the standard treatment of HER2+ Breast cancer: Efficacy in breast tumor and brain metastasis. *Small* **2022**, *18*, e2107550. [CrossRef] [PubMed]
111. Liu, H.-J.; Wang, M.; Shi, S.; Hu, X.; Xu, P. A Therapeutic sheep in metastatic wolf's clothing: Trojan Horse Approach for Cancer Brain Metastases Treatment. *Nanomicro Lett.* **2022**, *14*, 114. [CrossRef]
112. Birch-Machin, M.A. The role of mitochondria in ageing and carcinogenesis. *Clin. Exp. Dermatol.* **2006**, *31*, 548–552. [CrossRef] [PubMed]
113. Tokarz, P.; Blasiak, J. Role of mitochondria in carcinogenesis. *Acta Biochim. Pol.* **2014**, *61*, 671–678. [CrossRef] [PubMed]
114. Gazdar, A.F.; Bunn, P.A.; Minna, J.D. Small-cell lung cancer: What we know, what we need to know and the path forward. *Nat. Rev. Cancer* **2017**, *17*, 725–737, Erratum in *Nat. Rev. Cancer* **2017**, *17*, 765. [CrossRef] [PubMed]
115. Zhang, J.; Han, M.; Zhang, J.; Abdalla, M.; Sun, P.; Yang, Z.; Zhang, C.; Liu, Y.; Chen, C.; Jiang, X. Syphilis mimetic nanoparticles for cuproptosis-based synergistic cancer therapy via reprogramming copper metabolism. *Int. J. Pharm.* **2023**, *640*, 123025. [CrossRef]
116. Wang, Z.; Jin, D.; Zhou, S.; Dong, N.; Ji, Y.; An, P.; Wang, J.; Luo, Y.; Luo, J. Regulatory roles of copper metabolism and cuproptosis in human cancers. *Front. Oncol.* **2023**, *13*, 1123420. [CrossRef]
117. Hartwig, C.; Zlatic, S.A.; Wallin, M.; Vrailas-Mortimer, A.; Fahrni, C.J.; Faundez, V. Trafficking mechanisms of P-type ATPase copper transporters. *Curr. Opin. Cell Biol.* **2019**, *59*, 24–33. [CrossRef]
118. Xie, J.; Yang, Y.; Gao, Y.; He, J. Cuproptosis: Mechanisms and links with cancers. *Mol. Cancer* **2023**, *22*, 46. [CrossRef] [PubMed]
119. Tsvetkov, P.; Coy, S.; Petrova, B.; Dreishpoon, M.; Verma, A.; Abdusamad, M.; Rossen, J.; Joesch-Cohen, L.; Humeidi, R.; Spangler, R.D.; et al. Copper induces cell death by targeting lipoylated TCA cycle proteins. *Science* **2022**, *375*, 1254–1261. [CrossRef] [PubMed]
120. Kao, W.-C.A.; Pětrošová, H.; Ebady, R.; Lithgow, K.V.; Rojas, P.; Zhang, Y.; Kim, Y.-E.; Kim, Y.-R.; Odisho, T.; Gupta, N.; et al. Identification of Tp0751 (Pallilysin) as a Treponema pallidum Vascular Adhesin by Heterologous Expression in the Lyme disease Spirochete. *Sci. Rep.* **2017**, *7*, 1538. [CrossRef] [PubMed]
121. Todeschi, J.; Dannhoff, G.; Chibbaro, S.; Segbedji, F.; Spatola, G.; Mallereau, C.-H.; Noel, G.; Schott, R.; Lhermitte, B.; Cebula, H.; et al. Second Cancer affecting the central nervous system: Systematic literature review exploring the link between malignant melanoma and glioblastoma. *World Neurosurg.* **2023**, *179*, 178–184. [CrossRef]
122. Killela, P.J.; Reitman, Z.J.; Jiao, Y.; Bettegowda, C.; Agrawal, N.; Diaz, L.A.; Friedman, A.H.; Friedman, H.; Gallia, G.L.; Giovanella, B.C.; et al. TERT promoter mutations occur frequently in gliomas and a subset of tumors derived from cells with low rates of self-renewal. *Proc. Natl. Acad. Sci. USA* **2013**, *110*, 6021–6026. [CrossRef]
123. Nonoguchi, N.; Ohta, T.; Oh, J.-E.; Kim, Y.-H.; Kleihues, P.; Ohgaki, H. TERT promoter mutations in primary and secondary glioblastomas. *Acta Neuropathol.* **2013**, *126*, 931–937. [CrossRef] [PubMed]
124. Huang, F.W.; Hodis, E.; Xu, M.J.; Kryukov, G.V.; Chin, L.; Garraway, L.A. Highly recurrent TERT promoter mutations in human melanoma. *Science* **2013**, *339*, 957–959. [CrossRef] [PubMed]
125. Horn, S.; Figl, A.; Rachakonda, P.S.; Fischer, C.; Sucker, A.; Gast, A.; Kadel, S.; Moll, I.; Nagore, E.; Hemminki, K.; et al. TERT promoter mutations in familial and sporadic melanoma. *Science* **2013**, *339*, 959–961. [CrossRef]
126. Qi, F.; Yin, Z.; Wang, G.; Zeng, S. Clinical and Prognostic Significance of O6-Methylguanine-DNA Methyltransferase Promoter Methylation in Patients with Melanoma: A Systematic Meta-Analysis. *Ann. Dermatol.* **2018**, *30*, 129. [CrossRef] [PubMed]

127. Solomon, D.A.; Kim, J.-S.; Cronin, J.C.; Sibenaller, Z.; Ryken, T.; Rosenberg, S.A.; Ressom, H.; Jean, W.; Bigner, D.; Yan, H.; et al. Mutational inactivation of PTPRD in glioblastoma multiforme and malignant melanoma. *Cancer Res.* **2008**, *68*, 10300–10306. [CrossRef]
128. Schindler, G.; Capper, D.; Meyer, J.; Janzarik, W.; Omran, H.; Herold-Mende, C.; Schmieder, K.; Wesseling, P.; Mawrin, C.; Hasselblatt, M.; et al. Analysis of BRAF V600E mutation in 1,320 nervous system tumors reveals high mutation frequencies in pleomorphic xanthoastrocytoma, ganglioglioma and extra-cerebellar pilocytic astrocytoma. *Acta Neuropathol.* **2011**, *121*, 397–405. [CrossRef] [PubMed]
129. Davies, H.; Bignell, G.R.; Cox, C.; Stephens, P.; Edkins, S.; Clegg, S.; Teague, J.; Woffendin, H.; Garnett, M.J.; Bottomley, W.; et al. Mutations of the BRAF gene in human cancer. *Nature* **2002**, *417*, 949–954. [CrossRef]
130. Horbinski, C. ToBRAFoR Not ToBRAF: Is that even a question anymore? *J. Neuropathol. Exp. Neurol.* **2012**, *72*, 2–7. [CrossRef] [PubMed]
131. Scarbrough, P.M.; Akushevich, I.; Wrensch, M.; Il'yasova, D. Exploring the association between melanoma and glioma risks. *Ann. Epidemiol.* **2014**, *24*, 469–474. [CrossRef]
132. Sambade, M.; Deal, A.; Schorzman, A.; Luft, J.C.; Bowerman, C.; Chu, K.; Karginova, O.; Van Swearingen, A.; Zamboni, W.; DeSimone, J.; et al. Efficacy and Pharmacokinetics of a Modified acid-labile docetaxel-PRINT ® Nanoparticle Formulation Against non-small-cell Lung Cancer Brain Metastases. *Nanomedicine* **2016**, *11*, 1947–1955. [CrossRef] [PubMed]
133. Kim, D.H.; Choi, Y.J.; Sung, K.J.; Yoo, S.; Sung, Y.H.; Kim, J.K.; Choi, C.; Yun, M.; Lee, E.Y.; Jin, Y.S.; et al. Efficacy of nano-particulated, water-soluble erlotinib against intracranial metastases of EGFR-mutant lung cancer. *Mol. Oncol.* **2018**, *12*, 2182–2190. [CrossRef] [PubMed]
134. Negrini, S.; De Palma, R.; Filaci, G. Anti-cancer Immunotherapies Targeting Telomerase. *Cancers* **2020**, *12*, 2260. [CrossRef] [PubMed]
135. Qu, Z.; Dong, J.; Zhang, Z.Y. Protein tyrosine phosphatases as emerging targets for cancer immunotherapy. *Br. J. Pharmacol.* 2023; *early view*. [CrossRef]
136. Koya, R.C.; Mok, S.; Otte, N.; Blacketor, K.J.; Comin-Anduix, B.; Tumeh, P.C.; Minasyan, A.; Graham, N.A.; Graeber, T.G.; Chodon, T.; et al. BRAF inhibitor vemurafenib improves the antitumor activity of adoptive cell immunotherapy. *Cancer Res.* **2012**, *72*, 3928–3937. [CrossRef]
137. Kreuter, J.; Shamenkov, D.; Petrov, V.; Ramge, P.; Cychutek, K.; Koch-Brandt, C.; Alyautdin, R. Apolipoprotein-mediated transport of nanoparticle-bound drugs across the blood-brain barrier. *J. Drug Target.* **2002**, *10*, 317–325. [CrossRef]
138. Zhang, L.; Zhao, G.; Dalrymple, T.; Husiev, Y.; Bronkhorst, H.; Forn-Cuní, G.; Lopes-Bastos, B.; Snaar-Jagalska, E.; Bonnet, S. Cyclic Ruthenium-Peptide Prodrugs Penetrate the Blood-Brain Barrier and Attack Glioblastoma upon Light Activation in Orthotopic Zebrafish Tumor Models. *ACS Cent. Sci.* **2024**, *10*, 2294–2311. [CrossRef]
139. Yaremenko, A.V.; Khan, M.M.; Zhen, X.; Tang, Y.; Tao, W. Clinical advances of mRNA vaccines for cancer immunotherapy. *Med* **2025**, *6*, 100562. [CrossRef] [PubMed]
140. Cesarini, V.; Scopa, C.; Silvestris, D.A.; Scafidi, A.; Petrera, V.; Del Baldo, G.; Gallo, A. Aptamer-Based In Vivo Therapeutic Targeting of Glioblastoma. *Molecules* **2020**, *25*, 4267. [CrossRef]
141. Ni, K.; Lan, G.; Chan, C.; Quigley, B.; Lu, K.; Aung, T.; Guo, N.; La Riviere, P.; Weichselbaum, R.R.; Lin, W. Nanoscale metal-organic frameworks enhance radiotherapy to potentiate checkpoint blockade immunotherapy. *Nat. Commun.* **2018**, *9*, 2351. [CrossRef] [PubMed]
142. Dunn, G.P.; Bruce, A.T.; Ikeda, H.; Old, L.J.; Schreiber, R.D. Cancer immunoediting: From immunosurveillance to tumor escape. *Nat. Immunol.* **2002**, *3*, 991–998. [CrossRef] [PubMed]
143. Smyth, M.J.; Godfrey, D.I.; Trapani, J.A. A fresh look at tumor immunosurveillance and immunotherapy. *Nat. Immunol.* **2001**, *2*, 293–299. [CrossRef] [PubMed]
144. Gajewski, T.F.; Woo, S.-R.; Zha, Y.; Spaapen, R.; Zheng, Y.; Corrales, L.; Spranger, S. Cancer immunotherapy strategies based on overcoming barriers within the tumor microenvironment. *Curr. Opin. Immunol.* **2013**, *25*, 268–276. [CrossRef] [PubMed]
145. Joyce, J.A.; Fearon, D.T. T cell exclusion, immune privilege, and the tumor microenvironment. *Science* **2015**, *348*, 74–80. [CrossRef] [PubMed]
146. Schaue, D. A century of radiation therapy and adaptive immunity. *Front. Immunol.* **2017**, *8*, 431. [CrossRef]
147. Ganau, M.; Gallinaro, P.; Cebula, H.; Scibilia, A.; Todeschi, J.; Gubian, A.; Nannavecchia, B.; Signorelli, F.; Pop, R.; Coca, H.A.; et al. Intracranial Metastases from Prostate Carcinoma: Classification, Management, and Prognostication. *World Neurosurg.* **2020**, *134*, e559–e565. [CrossRef] [PubMed]
148. Kiess, A.P.; Wolchok, J.D.; Barker, C.A.; Postow, M.A.; Tabar, V.; Huse, J.T.; Chan, T.A.; Yamada, Y.; Beal, K. Stereotactic radiosurgery for melanoma brain metastases in patients receiving ipilimumab: Safety profile and efficacy of combined treatment. *Int. J. Radiat. Oncol. Biol. Phys.* **2015**, *92*, 368–375. [CrossRef] [PubMed]

149. Wang, Z.; Chen, F.; Cao, Y.; Zhang, F.; Sun, L.; Yang, C.; Xie, X.; Wu, Z.; Sun, M.; Ma, F.; et al. An Engineered Nanoplatform with Tropism Toward Irradiated Glioblastoma Augments Its Radioimmunotherapy Efficacy. *Adv. Mater.* **2024**, *36*, e2314197. [CrossRef] [PubMed]
150. Chen, M.-H.; Liu, T.-Y.; Chen, Y.-C.; Chen, M.-H. Combining Augmented Radiotherapy and Immunotherapy through a Nano-Gold and Bacterial Outer-Membrane Vesicle Complex for the Treatment of Glioblastoma. *Nanomaterials* **2021**, *11*, 1661. [CrossRef] [PubMed]
151. Liu, Y.; Zhang, P.; Li, F.; Jin, X.; Li, J.; Chen, W.; Li, Q. Metal-based NanoEnhancers for Future Radiotherapy: Radiosensitizing and synergistic effects on tumor cells. *Theranostics* **2018**, *8*, 1824–1849. [CrossRef]
152. Blezinger, P.; Wang, J.; Gondo, M.; Quezada, A.; Mehrens, D.; French, M.; Singhal, A.; Sullivan, S.; Rolland, A.; Ralston, R.; et al. Systemic Inhibition of Tumor Growth and Tumor Metastases by Intramuscular Administration of the Endostatin Gene. *Nat. Biotechnol.* **1999**, *17*, 343–348. [CrossRef]
153. Lu, L.; Chen, H.; Wang, L.; Zhao, L.; Cheng, Y.; Wang, A.; Wang, F.; Zhang, X. A Dual Receptor Targeting- and BBB Penetrating-Peptide Functionalized Polyethyleneimine Nanocomplex for Secretory Endostatin Gene Delivery to Malignant Glioma. *Int. J. Nanomed.* **2020**, *15*, 8875–8892. [CrossRef] [PubMed]
154. Simões, R.V.; Serganova, I.S.; Kruchevsky, N.; Leftin, A.; Shestov, A.A.; Thaler, H.T.; Sukenick, G.; Locasale, J.W.; Blasberg, R.G.; Koutcher, J.A.; et al. Metabolic plasticity of metastatic breast cancer cells: Adaptation to changes in the microenvironment. *Neoplasia* **2015**, *17*, 671–684. [CrossRef] [PubMed]
155. Himič, V.; Syrmos, N.; Ligarotti, G.K.I.; Ganau, M. Latest Insights on Genomic and Epigenomic Mechanisms of Nanotoxicity. In *Impact of Engineered Nanomaterials in Genomics and Epigenomics*; Sahu, S.C., Ed.; John Wiley & Sons, Inc.: Hoboken, NJ, USA, 2023. [CrossRef]

MDPI AG
Grosspeteranlage 5
4052 Basel
Switzerland
Tel.: +41 61 683 77 34

Brain Sciences Editorial Office
E-mail: brainsci@mdpi.com
www.mdpi.com/journal/brainsci

www.ingramcontent.com/pod-product-compliance
Lightning Source LLC
Chambersburg PA
CBHW062042220926
51850CB00010B/2636
9783725853397